MEDICINE TAKERS, PRESCRIBERS
AND HOARDERS

Reports of the Institute for Social Studies in Medical Care

The Institute for Social Studies in Medical Care was formed in 1970 as a development from the Institute of Community Studies, and its inauguration coincided with the publication by its Director Dr Ann Cartwright of *Parents and Family Planning Services*.

Further reports from the Institute for Social Studies in Medical Care will appear in this new series.

Medicine Takers, Prescribers and Hoarders
Karen Dunnell and Ann Cartwright

Life before Death
Ann Cartwright, Lisbeth Hockey and John L. Anderson

A catalogue of series of Social Science books published by Routledge will be found at the end of this volume.

MEDICINE TAKERS, PRESCRIBERS AND HOARDERS

KAREN DUNNELL
ANN CARTWRIGHT

LONDON AND BOSTON
ROUTLEDGE & KEGAN PAUL

First published 1972
by Routledge & Kegan Paul Ltd
Broadway House, 68–74 Carter Lane,
London EC4V 5EL and
9 Park Street,
Boston, Mass. 02108, U.S.A.
Printed in Great Britain by
Richard Clay (The Chaucer Press) Ltd
Bungay, Suffolk

Library of Congress Catalog Card Number: 72-85957
ISBN 0 7100 7351 8

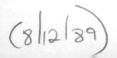
(8/12/89)

CONTENTS

Contents

ACKNOWLEDGMENTS

Many people have helped and contributed to this study:

The people and the general practitioners who answered the questions.

The Department of Health and Social Security and the Scottish Home and Health Department financed it and provided additional information about general practitioners.

The Social Survey Division of the Office of Population Censuses and Surveys lent us a sampling frame of parliamentary constituencies.

Queen Mary College, University of London, and the Institute of Computer Science let us use their machines and Margaret Manning at the University of London Computer Centre did some computing.

The interviewers: June Bathgate, Enid Binks, Elizabeth Blenman, Carol Chitty, Jil Cove, Janet Cummins, Joan Ellis, Connie Frost, Hilary Gellman, Flo Green, Cherry Knott, Vic Lanser, Ellen Latham, Jen Lazarus, Janet Martin, Muriel Toney, Annie Walker and Kay Young.

The coders: Anna Bender, Gwen Cartwright, Linda Clayton, Peter Evans, Nina Fishman, June Humphry, David McCarthy, Kate MacDonald, Martin Njeuma, Philip Osborn, Joanna Smart, Helen Ward and Hilary Wooder.

Joan Deane and Dorothy Hills punched the cards.

Jean Betteridge, Peter Quince, Heather Robertson, Wendy Smith and Jane Thomas helped in the preparation or analysis.

Philip Baldwin and David Sperlinger checked the report.

Wyn Tucker helped at all the early stages of the study and shared in the field work supervision.

John Anderson, Christine Fitz-Gerald, Hilary Lance, Peter Marris, Marjorie Waite and other colleagues helped in various ways.

Dr Roy Goulding and Susan McLean of the Poisons Unit at Guy's Hospital identified the tablets.

Acknowledgments

Jasper Woodcock created the classification of medicines and commented on the draft.

Those who have been or are working in the same field who gave advice, particularly T. H. Bewley, Dick Joyce, Len Ratoff, David Robinson, Nevil Silverton, Mike Wadsworth and Irv Zola.

Members of the Institute's Advisory Committee gave encouragement and advice throughout: Abe Adelstein, Maurice Backett, J. B. Cornish, John Fry, Austin Heady, Mike Heasman, John Horder, Margot Jefferys, John Reid, Michael Warren, Peter Willmott, John Wing and, more recently, Joyce Leeson.

We are indebted to all these and others who helped and contributed to the preliminary inquiries and to the main study.

INTRODUCTION

The consumption of medicines in Britain is increasing. In the five years between 1963 and 1968 the average number of prescriptions per person on National Health Service prescribing lists rose from 4·6 to 5·7 a year. The number of prescriptions rose from 206 millions to 267 millions, the annual cost from £96 million to £152 million.[1] When the National Health Service was introduced in 1948 and prescribed medicines became available free of charge to everyone, many people thought, and those in the patent[2] medicine industry feared, that people would buy fewer medicines over the counter. This did not happen and the retail sales of medicines increased and continued to do so,[3] in spite of new legislation and codes of practice controlling their advertising.[4] The pharmaceutical industry has expanded faster than most other industries in Britain recently. Board of Trade Output Indices for 1968 (at constant prices) show that the production of pharmaceutical preparations has increased by 67% since 1963, compared with an overall rise of 40% in the chemical industry and 21% in manufacturing industry as a whole.[5] Both the public and the medical profession are the targets of the industry's marketing policies. The industry has created an increasing supply of new products both for the ethical[6] and over-the-counter markets; the public and the doctors keep up the demand.

[1] These figures refer to prescriptions given by general practitioners. See *Annual Reports* of the Ministry of Health for the years 1963–7 and the *Annual Report* of the Department of Health and Social Security for the year 1968.
[2] Patent medicines or counter proprietary preparations are those which are advertised to the public and subject to purchase tax. Doctors are not allowed to prescribe them under the National Health Service.
[3] Office of Health Economics, 1968, *Without Prescription*, p. 4.
[4] Code of Advertising Practice Committee, 1970, *The British Code of Advertising Practice*.
[5] The Association of the British Pharmaceutical Industry, 1970, *The Pharmaceutical Industry and the Nation's Health*, fifth edition.
[6] Ethical preparations are those which are advertised only to the medical, dental

At the same time, the number of spells of certified sickness absence has also increased, and an analysis of this trend has shown that less serious illness is increasingly regarded as justification for absence from work. One conclusion drawn from the analysis was that 'at least part of the explanation for increased incapacity attributed to these . . . ("trivial") . . . conditions is a change in threshold levels at which an illness is translated into a spell of sickness absence'.[7]

But there is no evidence of an increase in the number of consultations with general practitioners.[8] The combination of these various trends suggests that an increasing proportion of general practitioner consultations result in a prescription, and people are turning more to self-medication than they used to do. There appears to have been a change not only in the threshold at which illness is seen as justifying sickness absence, but also in the level at which treatment is felt to be appropriate, and it is this which has led to an increase in the consumption of medicines.

Aims of the study

Questions raised by these changes which this study tries to answer fall into three broad groups. The first is concerned with the distribution and nature of medicine taking: who takes which sorts of medicines for what types of conditions and symptoms? The second is about the role of the medical profession: the relationship between professional treatment and self-medication, the ways in which doctors may encourage or discourage self-treatment, the frequency, nature and duration of repeat prescribing and the influence of doctors' views on their patients' medicine-taking behaviour. The third relates to the storage of medicines in people's homes: what medicines are kept, where and for how long?

But the basic aim of the study is wider and deeper than these specific questions. It is to illuminate the relationship between patients and doctors, and to find out more about the functioning of the health service. By looking at the self-treated symptoms

---

[7] Office of Health Economics, 1971, *Off Sick*, p. 16.
[8] Royal College of General Practitioners, 1970, *Present State and Future Needs of General Practice*.

---

and pharmaceutical professions, and not directly to the consumer. Most, but not all, are only obtainable with a doctor's prescription.

which people reported we get some idea of the hidden part of the iceberg of illness not brought to the attention of doctors. We can compare the people who seek different kinds of help. We can see how their personal characteristics and attitudes, and the inter-personal factors between patients and doctors, influence decisions about whether and where to look for help. The views of doctors on which conditions are appropriate for consultation show how they see some of the limits of their role. Variations between people in different social classes throw light on the distribution of care and the equity of services. In these sorts of ways this study of the people who take, and the doctors who prescribe, medicines can add to our understanding of health behaviour.

Methods

The study was done in fourteen parliamentary constituencies in Britain. These were Merton and Mordon (London), Woolwich–East (London), Swansea–West (Glamorgan), Canterbury (Kent), Liverpool–Walton (Lancashire), Southampton–Itchen (Hamp-shire), Knutsford (Cheshire), New Forest (Hampshire), Grimsby (Lincolnshire), West Dorset, South Worcestershire, Birmingham–Hall Green (Warwickshire), Glasgow–Shettleston (Lanarkshire) and West Lothian. They were selected, after stratification, with a probability proportional to the number of electors. The way this was done is described in Appendix I. Samples of adults, children, households and doctors were selected in the study areas.

For the *adults*, people aged 21 and over, 150 electors were chosen at random from each of the twelve constituencies in England and Wales and ninety from each of the two Scottish ones. This gave a total sample of 1,980 adults who were first approached between March and July 1969. Initially the response rate was low: 69% of people still living in the area. Other interviewers called back on those people who had not been contacted or who had refused. This procedure raised the response rate to 76%. Finally 1,412 adults were interviewed. Table 1 shows the reasons for failure. Twenty per cent finally refused and 4% were either not contacted, were too ill, old or deaf, or were in hospital. Appendix I compares the age and sex of the sample interviewed with data for the population. It was found that the sample had fewer young adults aged 21–24 and more older ones between 65 and 74 than

3

would be expected in a representative sample of the adult population. This probably reflects the availability of these two groups for interviewing.

TABLE I   *Response of the sample of adults*

	Number	Percentage of people still living in area
Interviewed	1,412	76
Refused	365	20
Too ill, deaf, senile	19	1
Temporarily away or not contacted for other reason	54	3
Died	32	—
Moved	98	—
Total	1,980	1,850 (= 100%)

A sample of 969 *households* was chosen from the original sample of adults.[9] The sample of *children* was made up of all those under 15 years living in these households. Information was obtained about the medicines kept in 686 of the chosen households (71%) and about 519 children.[10] No information was collected about people aged 15–20. It was not felt appropriate to question their parents about these late teenagers' medicine-taking habits and because of their mobility and ineligibility at the time for inclusion on the electoral register they would have been a difficult age-range to sample and locate for interview.

The sample of *doctors* was made up of the general practitioners of the adults who were interviewed.[11] Less than 1% did not have a doctor, 98% had one under the National Health Service and 1% had a private doctor. Many had the same doctors. Altogether they gave the names of 598 general practitioners. After the doctor's name was given at an interview he was sent a letter telling him about the study and asking him to help by answering a questionnaire at a later date. About a year later the doctors were sent a

[9] The way this was done is described in Appendix I.
[10] The number of children under 15 were ascertained in 90% of the 969 households. Information was obtained about 89% of the children who were identified. Details are given in Appendix I.
[11] Question 6: 'Who is your own doctor?' RECORD NAME, INITIALS AND ADDRESS. Question 7: 'Is that under the National Health Service or privately?'

4

letter, a summary of results from the study and a postal question-naire. After two reminders, 326 (56%) had replied. This response was very low, as pilot inquiries had suggested it might be. Additional information on the age, sex, type of practice and some prescribing costs of the doctors was obtained from the Department of Health and Social Security and the Scottish Home and Health Department. Full details of possible biases in the sample are given in Appendix II. Comparisons of those who replied with those who did not, show that the respondents tended to be younger than the others, but there was no evidence of any difference in their prescribing patterns.

Several methods of data collection were used. The adults were interviewed with a questionnaire about the medicines they had taken during the last twenty-four hours and during the two weeks before the interview, about the symptoms they had in that time and about their attitudes towards health, medicines and the medical profession in general (a copy of the questionnaire is in Appendix VIII). The mothers of the children were interviewed with a directly comparable questionnaire. People were asked about all consultations with a doctor and prescriptions received during the same two weeks.

To see whether people had prescriptions made up and whether they tried the medicines, all those who had been given a prescription in the two-week period were asked to complete a diary about all the medicines they took in the subsequent two weeks. Diary information was obtained for 73% of the total of 399 prescriptions.

Housewives were asked about all the medicines in the sample of households. Lists were made and questions asked about the use and storage of each one. As people are not always aware of the name or the content of drugs, especially prescribed ones, the interviewers collected samples of any tablets that were not identified by respondents, unless they were currently being taken. In addition a one-in-ten sample of all tablets, whether they were identified or not, was taken to see if they were really what people thought they were. The tablets collected were identified, where possible, by the Poisons Unit at Guy's Hospital, London.

These methods of sampling and the way in which the information has been collected, mainly through questionnaires, have a number of obvious limitations. Incomplete response may lead to bias and although we can identify some of these, and show that others do not exist, it is possible that there are others which we have not been able to pinpoint. In addition the questions asked may sometimes have been ambiguous or inappropriate and the answers inaccurate because of misunderstanding, poor recall, or even a wish to mislead or cover up. The ways in which answers have been grouped may over-simplify or occasionally distort people's views. For all these reasons the data needs to be interpreted with care: reported behaviour is not necessarily actual behaviour.

Themes

Chapter 2 is largely descriptive. It looks at the extent of medicine taking and the amount of reported ill health. Other studies have shown that most people experience some symptoms and take some medicine during a four-week period.[12] The prevalence of various symptoms and conditions are considered and the relationship between ill health and medicine taking discussed. Variations in illness behaviour with age and sex are looked at and comparisons made with a number of other studies.[13]

Chapter 3 describes in detail this common practice of medicine taking and analyses the association between self-medication and professional prescription. Results from a survey of a working-class housing estate in 1954–5[14] suggested that self-medication was not an alternative to professional consultation. Soon after this Kessel and Shepherd,[15] who compared non-attenders with recent attenders in a general practice, reached a similar conclusion. Our findings on the relation between medical consultation and self-medication are different.

The succeeding three chapters (4–6) are each concerned to some extent with the role played by general practitioners. Chapter 4 examines the extent and nature of repeat prescribing. Chapter 5

[12] Logan, W. P. D. and Brooke, E. M., 1957, *The Survey of Sickness, 1943–1952.* Wadsworth, M., Butterfield, W. J. H. and Blaney, R., 1971, *Health and Sickness: the Choice of Treatment.*
[13] Gray, P. G. and Cartwright, Ann, 1954. 'Who gets the medicine?'; also Logan and Brooke, op. cit., and Wadsworth *et al.*, op. cit.
[14] Jefferys, Margot, Brotherston, J. H. F. and Cartwright, Ann, 1960, 'Consumption of medicines on a working-class housing estate'.
[15] Kessel, N. and Shepherd, M., 1965, 'The health and attitudes of people who seldom consult a doctor'.

looks at the reliance and faith that people place in their doctors and how this relates to their medicine-taking habits. Chapter 6 is about the doctors' views of their role and their attitudes and practices in relation to prescribing. A number of studies have been concerned with differences in prescribing levels and have tried to explain these in various ways. Martin [16] collected information about prescriptions, doctors' practices, patients' social conditions, geographical location and morbidity arising in general practice in sixty-seven medium-sized county boroughs in 1951. Another paper [17] looked at differences between general practitioners and found that both higher educational qualifications and an orientation towards a 'whole person' view of the patient was associated with lower prescribing of drugs of all kinds. Our study takes rather different sorts of variables, mainly the views and medicine-taking practices of patients, and sees whether and how these relate to patterns of prescribing among general practitioners.

Chapter 7 is about medicines in the home. In 1965 a market research study [18] of the remedies people kept in their homes found that only 4% of them did not keep anything: most had analgesics. A scheme in Hartlepool [19] to recover unwanted prescribed medicines from peoples' homes produced over 43,000 tablets in one week. More than one-fifth of those identified were psychotropic [20] drugs. Our study details both the prescribed and non-prescribed medicines in people's homes, describes where they are kept and for how long and considers some of the implications of the medicine hoarding revealed.

The penultimate chapter (8) looks at the data from a different viewpoint and considers the patterns of consumption of the most commonly taken medicines. The final chapter draws together the findings from these different themes.

[16] Martin, J. P., 1957, *Social Aspects of Prescribing*.
[17] Joyce, C. R. B., Last, J. M. and Weatherall, M., 1968, 'Personal factors as a cause of differences in prescribing by general practitioners'.
[18] National Opinion Polls Ltd., 1965, *Home medication survey*.
[19] Nicholson, W. A., 1967, 'Collection of unwanted drugs from private homes'.
[20] Psychotropic drugs are defined here as hypnotics, tranquillisers, stimulants and appetite-suppressants and anti-depressives.

ILL HEALTH AND MEDICATION

This chapter starts by discussing people's perceptions of ill health and then goes on to describe the symptoms they reported. The decision about whether or not to take action about perceived illness and the selection of different lines of action are then considered. The chapter ends with a description of the age and sex variations of both symptom reporting and medication.

Perception of ill health

How many people feel healthy? We asked people whether they would describe their health in the two weeks before they were interviewed as excellent, good, fair or poor.[1] Just over a quarter of the adults said excellent, less than one in ten poor. The full distribution is shown in Table 2. More of the children, almost a half, were described as having excellent health; for one in twenty it was thought poor. And among the adults, health ratings were clearly related to age: the proportion describing their health as excellent declined from 35% of those under 35 to 17% of those aged 75 or over.

Earlier studies have shown that most people report some symptoms over a two- or four-week period. So feeling that one's health is excellent or good may not depend entirely on being free of symptoms. In this study only 9% of the adults, 37% of the children, were said not to have had any of a check list of symptoms during the previous two weeks.[2] Among the adults the average number of reported symptoms was 3·9. It was 6·2 among those

---

[1] Question 1: 'During the last two weeks—would you say your health has been excellent, good, fair or poor?'
[2] Question 20: 'I'd now like to ask you about things you might have had wrong with you in the last two weeks; What about . . .?' (For check list of symptoms see Table 4.)

who said their health had been poor but those who described it as excellent reported an average of 2·5 symptoms.

People's level of expectations, general sense of well-being, their views of their own health in relation to other people's, their view of their health in the last two weeks as compared with other times

TABLE 2   *Health rating by age*

Health in previous two weeks rated as:	Chil- dren under 15	Adults							All adults
		21–24	25–34	35–44	45–54	55–64	65–74	75+	
	%	%	%	%	%	%	%	%	%
Excellent	46	35	35	30	29	25	24	17	28
Good	37	34	38	40	44	35	41	30	39
Fair	12	26	19	22	22	28	26	30	24
Poor	5	5	8	8	5	12	9	23	9
Number of people (= 100%)ᵃ	519	81	230	289	266	257	190	84	1,401

ᵃ The numbers are slightly less than the total interviewed because some people did not answer all the questions. In other tables too, small numbers are excluded for the same reason.

and a general impression rather than a recollection of detail may all contribute to this apparent anomaly. But certainly most of those, five-sixths, who said their health was excellent reported some symptom. Only 4% of all adults had no symptoms and 'excellent' health, while less than 1% had fair or poor health but no symptoms in the previous two weeks. These few seemed to have either intermittent complaints which had not bothered them recently:

'Well I've been troubled with war wounds a long time but I've been O.K. in the last two weeks.'

or to be elderly:

'I am retired—take it easy—nice and steady.'

People who regarded themselves as healthy reported fewer symptoms than those who felt their health was fair or poor. Did they also report different sorts of symptoms? To look at this the distribution of different types of symptoms among people with the four health ratings were compared using as a base the total number of symptoms reported. Table 3 shows only the symptoms with a significant trend. Symptoms which increase with relative, as well as absolute, frequency with poor health rating are at the top. People who suffered from breathlessness, faintness or dizziness, loss of appetite, undue tiredness or a temperature were un-

TABLE 3   *Symptoms reported by adults with different health ratings*

| Percentage of all reported symptoms | Health in last two weeks rates as: | | | |
	excellent	good	fair	poor
	%	%	%	%
Breathlessness	2	4	4	5
Faintness or dizziness	1	2	2	4
Loss of appetite	1	1	2	3
Undue tiredness	2	4	5	5
Temperature	—	—	1	2
Headaches	14	10	9	7
Rashes, itches or other skin troubles	5	4	3	2
Burns, bruises, cuts or other accidents	4	3	1	1
Trouble with teeth or gums	3	2	2	1
Corns, bunions or any trouble with feet	6	6	4	4
Total symptoms reported (= 100%)	960	1,787	1,871	808
Average number of symptoms	2·5	3·4	5·6	6·2
Number of people	397	543	336	128

likely to think their health good. The symptoms reported relatively, but not absolutely, more often by those with good or excellent health were headaches, skin troubles, accidents and trouble with teeth or feet. These symptoms were not seen as incompatible with good health. To what extent are they the common symptoms?

Symptoms

The symptoms people were asked about, together with the proportion of adults and children who reported them, are shown in Table 4. The list consists almost entirely of symptoms. People

TABLE 4 *Symptoms reported by adults and children*

Symptom	Percentage reporting symptoms in a two-week period	
	Adults	Children
Sore throat	12	8
Breathlessness	15	1
Coughs, catarrh or phlegm	32	17
Cold, 'flu or running nose	18	18
Constipation	10	6
Diarrhoea	3	3
Vomiting	3	6
Indigestion	18	1
Eye strain or other eye trouble	14	4
Ear trouble	7	3
Faintness or dizziness	8	1
Headaches	38	8
Pain or trouble passing water	2	—
Loss of appetite	6	4
Any problem being under- or over-weight	10	—
Nerves, depression or irritability	21	3
Pains in the chest	5	—
Backache or pains in the back	21	1
Aches or pains in the joints, muscles, legs or arms	29	3
Palpitations or thumping heart	6	—
Piles	5	—
Sores or ulcers	4	2
Rashes, itches or other skin troubles	13	12
Sleeplessness	16	4
Swollen ankles	8	1
Burns, bruises, cuts or other accidents	9	16
Trouble with teeth or gums	7	12
Undue tiredness	16	2
Corns, bunions or any trouble with feet	19	2
Women's complaints [a]	5	1
A temperature	2	3
Any other symptoms	6	3
Number of people (= 100%)	1,410	519
Average number of symptoms reported	3·9	1·4

[a] Only asked of women and girls over 10 years old.

were not asked to make diagnoses.[3] The symptom most commonly reported by adults was headache. Nearly two-fifths of them had a headache during the two-week period. Next most common was coughs, catarrh or phlegm, then aches or pains in the muscles or joints and after that backache and nerves, depression or irritability. So among the five most common symptoms only headache was mentioned relatively frequently among those with good health. Foot troubles were mentioned by a fifth of adults. In another study,[4] focused on trouble with feet, a quarter of the adults mentioned foot conditions spontaneously but another third, who at first said they had no foot problems, reported some when asked about a specific list. Foot troubles are therefore probably more common than our figure suggests and this may be why they are accepted as compatible with good health. But it is also possible that the prevalence of other symptoms is under-estimated; the more specifically symptoms are described at an interview the more people will report them. Kosa *et al.*[5] found that a daily recording of health events for a seven-day period yielded about 12% more episodes than a structured seven-day recall.

Skin troubles, accidents, trouble with feet and teeth—the other symptoms apart from headaches reported relatively frequently by the healthy—are all relatively peripheral or external. Because of this they may be regarded as not threatening. For much of the time people may be unaware of them or regard them as discomforts: they do not 'feel sick'. For these reasons the awareness of a symptom can exist without the recognition or acceptance of ill health.

Action

Taking action about a particular symptom or about a generalised feeling of malaise depends first on the recognition that something is abnormal or wrong, then on the decision that it is appropriate to do something about it. This decision may depend not only on a belief or hope that something can be done to relieve or cure the

[3] For a discussion about this see Cartwright, Ann, 1959, 'Some problems in the collection and analysis of morbidity data obtained from sample surveys'.
[4] Clarke, May, 1969, *Trouble with Feet*, p. 13.
[5] Kosa, J., Alpert, J. J. and Haggerty, R. J., 1967, 'On the reliability of family health information. A comparative study of mothers' reports on illness and related behaviour'.

symptom, but may also be a way of justifying the adoption of the sick role and an indication that the person is attempting to get well. Decisions, or a series of decisions, have then to be made about the choice of action. People may consult their general practitioner, take over-the-counter medicines, seek the help of such people as chiropodists, herbalists or osteopaths or ask for the advice of their relatives and friends.[6]

Several studies have shown that people decide to obtain medical care from their general practitioner or a hospital for only a small proportion of their complaints. The Survey of Sickness[7] found that less than a quarter of those complaining of illness had seen a doctor about the complaint. Horder and Horder[8] reported that in their general practice only a third of illnesses reached any medical agency. This proportion was confirmed by a survey in Bermondsey and Southwark.[9]

The present study substantiates that there is a large 'iceberg' of illness in the general population at any one time which is not known to the medical profession. Although 91% of the adults reported symptoms during the two weeks before interview only 16% had consulted a doctor during that time and 28% of the adults said they had not consulted their general practitioner at all during the previous twelve-month period. Medicine taking was a much more frequent form of action.

More than half the adults, 55%, said they had taken or used some medicine during the twenty-four hours before the interview. During the two weeks before the interview they had taken an average of 2·2 different items.[10] The distribution for adults and children is given in Table 5. Other studies found similar results. A survey of a working-class housing estate in 1954–5[11] showed that more than three-quarters of adults had taken or used some

---

[6] This is a very brief outline of the processes involved. For a detailed discussion see Robinson, David, 1971, *The Process of Becoming Ill*, pp. 21–37.
[7] Stocks, P., 1949, *Sickness in the Population of England and Wales in 1944–47*, p. 24.
[8] Horder, J. and Horder, E., 1954, 'Illness in general practice'.
[9] Wadsworth, M. E. J., Butterfield, W. J. and Blaney, R., 1971, *Health and Sickness: the Choice of Treatment*.
[10] Throughout the report when different numbers of medicines are discussed it is the number of different items that is being referred to. An item is a brand of medicine, so for example if someone had taken one brand of pain-killer for headache and another for arthritis, they would be coded as having taken two items of medicine.
[11] Jefferys, Margot, Brotherston, J. H. F. and Cartwright, Ann, 1960, 'Consumption of medicines on a working-class housing estate'.

kind of medicine during a four-week period. Ten years later a similar proportion of people in Bermondsey and Southwark (see note 9) were found to have taken medicines during a two-week period. These studies found that self-medication was more common than professional treatment. On this study too for every

TABLE 5 *Numbers of medicines taken by adults and children during a two-week period*

	Adults	Children
Proportion taking:	%	%
none	20	45
one	24	26
two	21	13
three	14	10
four	8	3
five	6	2
six or more	7	1
Mean number taken	2·2	1·1
Number of people (= 100%)	1,412	519

prescribed item taken in the two weeks there were two non-prescribed items. During the two weeks two-fifths of the adults had taken something prescribed, two-thirds something non-prescribed. One-fifth of the children had taken a prescribed medicine, nearly half a non-prescribed one.

The number of different items of medicine people had taken was correlated with the number of symptoms they reported for the two-week period. (Correlation coefficient for the adults was +0·60). Those adults reporting one symptom had taken an average of 1·1 medicines, those reporting six or more an average of 4·0. Some medicines were taken for preventive purposes; a fifth of those reporting no symptoms had taken or used at least one item of medicine. But in general people reported more symptoms than they reported medicines taken. No medicines were taken for almost half, 47%, of the reported symptoms.[12] Symptoms for

[12] Medicines taken for conditions said to be related to the symptoms have been included here as medication for that symptom.

which people were most likely to take medicines were a temperature, 94% had done so, headaches 83%, indigestion 81% and sore throats 78%. The sorts of medicines people take are considered in the next chapter. Before that the associations between the amount of medication, perception of ill health and age and sex are described.

Age variations

Earlier we saw that the proportion of people describing their health as excellent declined with increasing age. But rather surprisingly there was no clear trend with age in the number of symptoms reported although those aged 65 or more reported slightly more symptoms than those under 65: 4·3 compared with 3·8. This may be because as people get older they have a higher threshold of symptom acceptance. The average number of symptoms has been used as a crude index of ill health. But of course symptoms differ in their severity and the associated incapacity; they may be continuous or intermittent and if a person has a single severe symptom he may disregard other minor ones. Older people may report more severe symptoms. Certainly when the number of symptoms was held constant older people were less likely than younger ones to regard their health as excellent. This can be seen from Table 6. But the number of symptoms reported by those who felt their health excellent was similar for old and

TABLE 6   *Health rating, number of symptoms and age*

Number of symptoms reported:	Proportion reporting health excellent	
	Under 65 years	*65 years or more*
None	55% (98)	45% (20)
One	46% (192)	38% (37)
Two	35% (190)	29% (41)
Three	29% (142)	21% (38)
Four	28% (133)	23% (35)
Five or six	19% (172)	8% (39)
Seven or more	9% (196)	8% (63)

The figures in brackets are the numbers on which the percentages are based (= 1000%).

TABLE 7 *Variation in symptoms reported with age*

	Age group							All adults
	21–24	25–34	35–44	45–54	55–64	65–74	75+	
Percentage of adults reporting:	%	%	%	%	%	%	%	%
Sore throat	17	17	15	14	9	5	5	12
Breathlessness	5	8	12	17	20	22	19	15
Coughs, catarrh or phlegm	27	27	34	30	34	35	35	32
Cold, 'flu or running nose	25	23	19	17	15	15	15	18
Constipation	12	7	8	9	9	14	20	10
Diarrhoea	5	4	2	2	2	4	3	3
Vomiting	4	5	2	2	3	3	6	3
Indigestion	15	10	15	18	22	25	20	18
Eye strain	20	11	11	14	14	16	22	14
Ear trouble	4	3	6	6	5	17	13	7
Faintness or dizziness	6	7	7	6	7	12	14	8
Headaches	41	51	48	42	29	23	21	38
Pain or trouble passing water	—	—	—	2	2	3	6	2
Loss of appetite	9	4	4	7	6	6	6	6
Any problem being under- or overweight	16	7	11	14	9	9	8	11
Nerves, depression or irritability	27	27	24	22	16	13	19	21
Pains in the chest	5	4	4	6	6	9	3	5
Backache or pains in the back	21	17	22	21	21	23	17	21
Aches or pains in the joints, muscles, legs or arms	21	20	23	29	34	39	45	29
Palpitations or thumping heart	1	5	4	7	6	11	3	6
Piles	5	4	2	6	5	6	6	5
Sores or ulcers	5	4	4	3	2	4	8	4
Rashes, itches or other skin troubles	22	17	13	17	7	10	6	13
Sleeplessness	11	10	12	16	22	21	23	16
Swollen ankles	1	3	5	8	10	13	20	8
Burns, bruises, cuts or other accidents	14	11	9	12	9	2	3	9
Trouble with teeth or gums	12	8	10	5	6	5	3	7
Undue tiredness	17	16	19	15	17	12	15	16
Corns, bunions or any trouble with feet	17	13	10	15	23	35	33	19
Women's complaints like period pain[a]	23	18	12	14	2	1	—	10
	(47)	(123)	(141)	(138)	(139)	(106)	(54)	(748)
A temperature	2	3	2	4	1	—	—	2
Any other symptoms not already mentioned	6	6	4	5	5	8	10	6
Number of adults (= 100%)	81	230	289	269	258	194	86	1,410

[a] The figures in brackets are the numbers of women from which percentages were calculated.

young people. Older people reported rather different symptoms. They reported more breathlessness, constipation, indigestion, ear trouble, faintness, muscle and joint pains, sleeplessness, foot troubles and swollen ankles. Headaches, sore throats, nerves, rashes, accidents, women's complaints and trouble with teeth were more often reported by younger than older people (see Table 7).

The number of medicines taken was related to age in rather the same way as the total number of symptoms reported: those aged 65 or more took rather more medicines than those under 65 and there was little or no variation with age among those under 65. But the proportion taking any medicine increased with age and this trend was due to an increase in the proportion taking prescribed medicines. Table 8 gives these figures. The proportion

TABLE 8 *Variation in medicine taking with age*

Proportion who had taken:	Age group							All adults
	21–24	25–34	35–44	45–54	55–64	65–74	75 or more	
Any medicine	75%	80%	80%	78%	80%	82%	92%	80%
Prescribed medicine	33%	40%	36%	32%	43%	49%	71%	41%
Non-prescribed medicine	67%	69%	71%	67%	64%	65%	71%	67%
Average number of medicines taken	2·1	2·0	2·1	2·1	2·2	2·7	3·2	2·2
Number of adults (= 100%)	81	230	289	269	258	194	87	1,412
Average number of medicines taken by those who had taken some	2·8	2·5	2·6	2·7	2·7	3·3	3·5	2·7

taking any non-prescribed medicines did not vary with age. Neither did the proportion taking medicines for their symptoms. So far we have been looking at age differences among the adults. How did the children fit into the picture?

Children

For children the age trend was reversed. More symptoms were reported for younger than for older children, the health rating was less good for the younger children and they more often took both prescribed and non-prescribed medicines. This is shown in Table 9. Three-quarters of the children under 2 had been given non-prescribed medicines and this proportion fell to just over a third of those aged 10–14. We can only speculate about those aged 15–20. Between 10 and 14 the average number of reported

TABLE 9   *Variations with children's age*

	Age group				All children
	Under 2	*2–4*	*5–9*	*10–14*	
Health rating:	%	%	%	%	%
Excellent	38	49	44	50	46
Good	32	33	42	38	37
Fair	19	12	10	9	12
Poor	11	6	4	3	5
Average number of symptoms reported	2·1	1·6	1·3	1·2	1·4
Proportion who had taken:					
Any medicine	78%	65%	49%	46%	55%
Prescribed medicine	35%	21%	16%	16%	20%
Non-prescribed medicine	74%	55%	43%	37%	48%
Average number of medicines taken	2·0	1·3	0·9	0·8	1·1
Number of children (= 100%)	68	113	169	169	519

symptoms was 1·2, for those aged 21–24 it was 4·2 and the proportion taking non-prescribed medicines was 37% for those aged 10–14, 67% for those 21–24.[13] At what point in these six years is the downward trend among the children so dramatically reversed? A study which included adolescents aged 16–20, who were interviewed personally, found that foot trouble was almost as prevalent among the adolescents as among the adults.[14] This

[13] Part of this difference may arise because those aged 21–24 were interviewed personally. Information about those aged 10–14 was obtained from the children's mother who was also sometimes asked about her own health and health behaviour and about any other children. See Cartwright, Ann, 1957, 'The effect of obtaining information from different informants on a family morbidity inquiry'.
[14] Clarke, May, op. cit., p. 68.

finding and the size of the gap between the 10–14 and 21–24-year-olds suggest that the upward swing towards more symptoms and more medicine taking may start in the younger part of the 15–20 range. It may start at different ages for boys and girls.

Sex differences

The average number of symptoms reported for boys and girls was similar and there was no difference in the proportion of boys and girls who had been given non-prescribed medicines. Boys however, were more likely than girls to have been given prescribed medicines: 24% compared with 15%. This difference occurred within each of the four age groups. This finding is consistent with others which have reported the well-known tendency for male children to be more prone to illness and death than female children.[15] Sex differences among the adults were mainly in the opposite direction. Women reported more symptoms than men, an average of 4·5 each compared with 3·2. Table 10 shows that

TABLE 10   *Relationship between age, sex and the number of reported symptoms in adults*

	Mean number of reported symptoms							
	Age group							All ages
	21–24	25–34	35–44	45–54	55–64	65–74	75+	
Men	4·1 (34)	2·8 (107)	3·1 (148)	3·5 (131)	3·0 (119)	3·5 (88)	3·7 (33)	3·2 (661)
Women	4·2 (47)	4·4 (123)	4·4 (141)	4·4 (138)	4·4 (139)	4·9 (106)	4·7 (53)	4·5 (749)
All adults	4·2 (81)	3·7 (230)	3·7 (289)	4·0 (269)	3·8 (258)	4·2 (194)	4·3 (86)	3·9 (1,410)

The figures in brackets refer to the number of adults for whom the means were calculated.

there was a substantial difference between the sexes at all ages except those aged 21 to 24 years. The sorts of symptoms more often reported by women than men were constipation, faintness, headaches, weight problems, nerves, backache, muscle and joint

[15] Douglas, J. W. B. and Blomfield, J. M., 1958, *Children under Five*, p. 93.

pains, palpitations, sleeplessness, swollen ankles, undue tiredness and foot troubles. The only one reported more by men was coughs, catarrh or phlegm (see Table 11).

Women were also larger consumers of medicines than men. This difference was found in all age groups. More women than men

TABLE 11 *Variation with sex in reported symptoms*

	Men	Women
Percentage reporting:	%	%
Sore throat	11	13
Breathlessness	13	17
Coughs, catarrh or phlegm	35	29
Cold, 'flu or running nose	18	19
Constipation	6	14
Diarrhoea	2	4
Vomiting	3	3
Indigestion	16	19
Eye strain	13	15
Ear trouble	8	7
Faintness or dizziness	6	10
Headaches	30	46
Pain or trouble passing water	1	2
Loss of appetite	5	6
Any problem being under- or over-weight	7	14
Nerves, depression or irritability	14	27
Pains in the chest	6	5
Backache or pains in the back	18	23
Aches or pains in the joints, muscles, legs or arms	26	32
Palpitations or thumping heart	4	8
Piles	3	6
Sores or ulcers	3	5
Rashes, itches or other skin troubles	12	14
Sleeplessness	12	20
Swollen ankles	2	13
Burns, bruises, cuts or other accidents	9	9
Trouble with teeth or gums	6	8
Undue tiredness	10	21
Corns, bunions or any trouble with feet	15	23
Women's complaints like period pain	—	10
A temperature	3	2
Any other symptoms not already mentioned	6	5
Number of adults (= 100%)	661	749

had taken medicine during the two weeks asked about, also those women who had taken some medicine took more items than the men who had done so. Only 14% of the women had not taken or used any medicine, compared with nearly twice as many men, 27%. Half the women had taken something prescribed compared with less than a third of the men. Three-quarters of the women had taken some self-prescribed medicine, three-fifths of the men.[16] Women did not take more medicines just because they had more symptoms; they were more likely to take medicines for their symptoms. Table 12 shows that for the same number of symptoms women were more likely than men to take prescribed medicines. Differences in the taking of non-prescribed medicines were smaller but generally in the same direction.

TABLE 12   *Sex, symptoms and medicine taking*

Number of symptoms:	Proportion taking any prescribed medicine		Proportion taking any non-prescribed medicine	
	Men	*Women*	*Men*	*Women*
None	8% (79)	15% (41)	11% (79)	12% (41)
One	22% (125)	37% (104)	53% (125)	47% (104)
Two	29% (119)	40% (113)	59% (119)	72% (113)
Three	37% (92)	46% (90)	61% (92)	77% (90)
Four	26% (77)	45% (92)	74% (77)	81% (92)
Five	42% (57)	57% (67)	82% (57)	84% (67)
Six or more	54% (112)	68% (239)	85% (112)	88% (239)

The figures in brackets are the bases from which percentages were calculated (= 100%).

One possible explanation for women's higher consumption of non-prescribed medicines is that they generally take responsibility for the family shopping. They will therefore be exposed to the displays and advertising of remedies in shops. This may make them more likely to buy over-the-counter medicines for their symptoms. In addition women spend more time than men in the home, and the average household, as Chapter 7 will show, has

[16] As shown in the next chapter, 6% of all women were taking contraceptive pills. If this form of medicine taking is excluded, the proportion of women who were not taking any (other) medicines was 15% and the proportion taking prescribed medicines was 46%.

ten different items of medicine in it. In short, medicines may be more readily available to women and they may more often be made aware of them. These practical reasons may contribute to women's greater tendency to take medicine.

Summary

Most adults, two-thirds, regarded their health as excellent or good. At the same time the majority reported at least one symptom during a two-week period. The most frequently reported symptom, headache, was quite commonly reported by those who felt their health was good. Other symptoms reported relatively often by the healthy were accidents and 'external' complaints. These may have been accepted as not affecting people's health because they were not felt to be part of them.

Although many people felt healthy in spite of their symptoms they still recognised that something was wrong and attempted to do something about it. Four-fifths of the adults had taken or used some medicine in the two weeks before they were interviewed. The proportion of adults taking prescribed medicines increased with age but there was no variation in the extent of self-medication. Women had taken more of both kinds of medicine than men and this was not just a reflection of the greater number of symptoms they reported—they were more likely to take medicines for their symptoms. Self-prescribed medicines outnumbered prescribed ones by two to one. The next chapter looks in more detail at this medication.

THE NATURE OF MEDICATION

What sorts of medicines do people take? This is the basic question considered in this chapter. To answer it medicines are classified in two ways as well as by whether they were prescribed or not. The relationship between prescribed and non-prescribed medication is then examined.

Types of medicine

We asked people about the different sorts of medicines listed in Table 13. In drawing up this list a number of requirements were taken into account. We wanted it to be as comprehensive as possible so that it would make people think of all the various things they might have used. At the same time we did not want it to be too long, partly because it had to be read out twice—once when people were asked about the last twenty-four hours and again when they were asked about the last two weeks. Also the medicines had to be described in familiar terms which people would recognise. The list is a combination of medicines used with a particular intention such as 'indigestion remedies', 'anti-depressives, stimulants and pep-pills' and 'slimming aids'; medicines used on particular parts of the body or in particular ways such as 'gargles or mouth washes', 'suppositories' and 'eye drops, lotions or ointments'; and medicines with a specified content such as 'vitamin tablets'. The proportions of adults and children who had taken each kind of medicine during the two periods are shown in Table 13. Pain-killers were the type of medicine most often taken by adults. Forty-one per cent had taken them in the two weeks before the interview compared with 14% who had taken or used the next two most popular types: indigestion remedies and skin ointments or antiseptics. Thirteen per cent of the adults had taken throat or cough remedies, 4% cold or congestion

TABLE 13   *Proportions of adults and children taking different sorts of medicines during a 24-hour and two-week period*

Type of medicine	Adults		Children	
	Taken in last 24 hours	Taken in last two weeks	Taken in last 24 hours	Taken in last two weeks
	%	%	%	%
Gargles or mouthwashes	2	5	—	—
Health salts	3	8	1	3
Indigestion remedies	5	14	2	3
Laxatives	4	9	1	3
Suppositories	—	1	—	—
Throat or cough medicines or sweets	6	13	4	12
Cold or congestion relievers	2	4	1	4
Aspirin or other pain-killers	14	41	5	18
Sedatives, sleeping tablets, tranquillisers	8	10	1	2
Anti-depressives, stimulants, pep pills	1	1	—	—
Skin ointments, antiseptics	8	14	10	19
Eye drops, lotions, ointments	2	4	1	2
Embrocation or ointment to rub in	2	7	1	2
Inhalants, drops or things to sniff	3	4	1	2
Diarrhoea remedies	—	1	—	1
Corn pads, foot powders, creams or dressings	3	7	—	1
Tonics, rejuvenators	3	5	2	2
Slimming aids	1	1	—	—
Vitamin tablets	5	6	5	6
Medicinal foods	3	4	3	4
Surgical clothing, trusses, bandages, elastic stockings	6	8	1	3
Alcohol—for medicinal purposes [a]	2	4	—	—
Hormones (or contraceptive pills) [a]	3	4	—	—
Travel or other kind of sickness pills	—	1	—	2
Other	16	22	6	10
Number of people (= 100%)	1,412	1,412	519	519

[a] These were not included on the children's check list, contraceptive pills were only asked about if the informant was a woman.

relievers. A tenth had taken some kind of sedative in the two-week period and over 1% anti-depressives. One in ten of the women aged between 21 and 54 were taking oral contraceptives.

Children had a different pattern of use. Skin ointments and antiseptics were the medicines most used by children; a fifth had used one or more kinds during the two-week period, a tenth during the twenty-four hours before the interview. Nearly as many, 18%, had been given analgesics[1] during the two weeks. Twelve per cent of the children had taken throat or cough medicines, 6% vitamin tablets, 4% medicinal food and 4% cold or congestion relievers. All the other medicines asked about had been taken by 3% or less of the children. Just over a fifth of the adults and a tenth of the children had taken some medicine which they did not fit into the list. These included a relatively high proportion, 88%, of prescribed medicines against 26% for the classified ones. Some of these others were identified as such specific things as antibiotics, insulin, iron, digatalis and diuretics. Thirty-eight per cent of them could not be identified when the medicines were classified in a more pharmacological way based on respondents' descriptions of the medicines they had taken.[2]

Pharmacological classification

This was derived from the most commonly consulted index of prescribed branded medicines, the 'Monthly Index of Medical Specialities' (MIMS). This classifies medicines by the body systems upon which they are reputed to act, and within each system by the reputed effect of the medicine. This principle turned out to be equally applicable to over-the-counter remedies, so long as 'reputation' was interpreted historically rather than in the light of current pharmacological concepts. Table 14 shows the groups with their codes.[3] This classification enables us not

---

[1] Analgesics and antipyretics are medicines, the most common example being aspirin, which relieve pain and reduce body temperature.
[2] Question 9a: 'What was it? Has it a brand name? What's in it?'
[3] This classification was devised for the study by Jasper Woodcock who has done similar work in the Department of Pharmacology at the London Hospital Medical School. He is presently information officer at the Institute for the Study of Drug Dependence. The source of information used to establish the reputed effects of un-branded drugs (prescribed or not) and branded over-the-counter medicines was Todd, R. G., 1967, *Extra Pharmacopoeia Martindale*.

The Nature of Medication

TABLE 14 *The distributions of items of medicines taken by the adults and children in a two-week period within the pharmacological classification*

Pharmacological classification:			Adults %	Children %
01	S	Analgesics and antipyretics	20·0	18·2
02	L	Skin creams, balms, oils, powders, anti-pruritics, anaesthetics	3·1	11·3
03	L	Counter-irritants, embrocations, rubs	2·5	1·1
04	L	Mouth and throat preparations	4·2	4·1
05	S	Cough and lower respiratory preparations	4·1	8·5
06	S	Antacids, indigestion remedies	6·4	4·8
07	L	Sticking plasters, bandages, corn pads, dressings, poultices	3·4	3·0
08	S	Laxatives, health salts	7·4	4·8
19	S	Tonics	0·7	1·2
10	S	Iron, vitamin, mineral preparations	5·5	8·5
1X	S	Slimming preparations	0·3	—
1Y	S	Other nutritional and metabolic preparations	1·2	0·7
29	L	Eye preparations	1·7	1·1
20	L	Ear preparations	0·2	0·9
2X	L	Upper respiratory and nose preparations	2·0	3·0
2Y	S	Antihistamines, cold remedies	0·5	0·9
39	S	Sedatives, sleeping pills, tranquillisers	4·8	1·1
30	S	Antidepressants, stimulants	0·5	—
3X	S	Antinauseants, travel sickness preparations	0·2	1·9
3Y	S	Other drugs acting on the central nervous system	0·3	0·3
49	L	Antibiotic, antiseptic, fungicidal, keratolytic ointments and powders	2·3	4·8
40	L	Barrier creams, insect repellent creams, suntan lotions	0·3	—
4X	L	General antiseptics, germicides, disinfectants, cleaners	2·1	2·3
4Y	L	Corticosteroid skin preparations	1·7	2·8
59	S	Anti-rheumatic preparations, corticosteroids	0·6	0·2
50	S	Hormones	0·2	—
5X	S	Contraceptive pills	1·5	—
5Y	S	Genito-urinary preparations	0·9	—
69	L	Suppositories, rectal preparations	0·5	—
60	S	Anti-diarrhoea preparations	0·3	0·3
6X	S	Cardio-vascular preparations	1·4	—
6Y	S	Antibiotics, anti-infective agents, anthelmintics	1·1	4·4
79	S & L	Ordinary food and drinks used medicinally (e.g. alcohol, honey)	4·9	3·2
70	S	Diet	0·3	—
7X	S	Herbal remedies	0·1	—
89	L	Surgical clothing, trusses, appliances, elastic stockings	2·1	0·3
8X	S & L	Others (not elsewhere classifiable)	0·1	—
XX		Name of preparation untraceable	0·9	—
XY		Insufficient detail to classify preparation	9·6	6·3
		Total number of medicines (= 100%)	3,163	566

Groups prefixed S refer to medicines taken internally; groups prefixed L refer to medicines applied locally.

only to look at the medicines people took in a more precise way but also to make comparisons with data from other sources. In addition we can see the extent to which people's initial descriptions of their medicines in response to our check list tallies with this classification. This comparison reveals two types of error. For example the group who said they had taken aspirin or other pain-killers includes a few people whose analgesics were in fact something else, while those who had taken pain-killers but reported them for instance as cold remedies or other medicines, are excluded. This means not only that the estimated proportion of people taking aspirins is slightly wrong but also the characteristics of the people will be slightly different. Details are discussed in Appendix III. The errors are small and have been ignored in the analyses.

A comparison with data from the Department of Health and Social Security relating to dispensed prescriptions during 1968 is made in Table 15. To do this some of the thirty-nine groups from our pharmacological classification have been combined and the medicines taken by adults and children added together.[4] There is fairly reasonable agreement between the Department's figures and the distribution of prescribed medicines taken by the sample of adults and children in the two weeks before the interview.

Prescribed and non-prescribed medicines

Table 15 also shows that prescribed and non-prescribed medicines differed greatly in their therapeutic groups. The most common non-prescribed medicines were analgesics and antipyretics and ones for the digestive system. Nearly half the non-prescribed ones were in these two groups, less than a fifth of the prescribed ones. This variation reflects the difference in the availability of different kinds of medicines. Most of the drugs acting on the cardio-vascular, gentio-urinary and central nervous systems, those taken internally for infections and those affecting metabolism and allergic reactions are obtainable only on a doctor's prescription. These groups represent more than half of the prescribed medicines. Many of the medicines in the other therapeutic groups are more readily available to the public because they can be bought over-the-counter as well as obtained on prescription. The proportions

4 For a justification of this see Appendix I.

The Nature of Medication

TABLE 15 *A comparison of the medicines reported on the survey with prescriptions dispensed by chemists, drug stores and appliance contractors during 1968*

Therapeutic group (D.H.S.S.)	Prescriptions dispensed from chemists etc.[a]	Prescribed medicines taken by sample	Non-prescribed medicines taken by sample	All medicines taken by sample
	%	%	%	%
Preparations acting on the digestive system (06, 08, 19, 60, 69)	8·1	8·4	19·4	16·2
Preparations acting on the cardio-vascular and genito-urinary systems and diuretics (6X, 5y)	8·3	7·2	0·2	2·2
Preparations acting on the lower respiratory system (05)	11·0	7·8	4·2	5·3
Preparations acting on the nervous system:				
Analgesics and antipyretics (01)	7·5	6·8	28·0	21·8
Acting on CNS (30, 39, 3X, 3y)	20·5	18·6	0·9	6·1
Preparations acting systemically on infections and immunological preparations (6y)	13·9	6·0	—	1·8
Preparations affecting metabolism, nutrition and blood (10, 1X, 1y, 50, 5X)	8·6	17·4	6·9	9·9
Preparations used in rheumatic diseases (03, 59)	2·4	3·4	3·1	3·2
Preparations affecting allergic reactions (2y)	2·6	1·2	0·3	0·6
Preparations acting on ear, nose and throat (04, 20, 2X)	3·4	4·2	8·6	7·3
Preparations acting on the eye (29)	1·4	1·9	1·7	1·8
Preparations acting on the skin (02, 49, 40, 4X, 4y)	7·0	10·2	13·4	12·4
Medicinal food, drink, etc. (79, 70, 7X)	—	—	7·9	5·6
Dressings and appliances (89, 07)	3·0	6·5	5·4	5·7
Other (8X)	2·3	0·4	—	0·1
Total number of identified items (= 100%)	267·4 millions	985	2,375	3,360

Figures in brackets are the code numbers assigned to groups of medicines in the pharmacological classification.

[a] Figures obtained from Department of Health and Social Security, *Annual Report for 1968*. Prescriptions dispensed by dispensing general practitioners are excluded.

28

TABLE 16   *Proportions of different kinds of medicines which were prescribed by a doctor*

Pharmacological classification:	Adults' medicines	Children's medicines	Adults' and children's medicines
Analgesics and antipyretics	10% (631)	5% (103)	9% (734)
Skin creams, balms, oils, powders, anti-pruritics, anaesthetics	9% (97)	11% (64)	10% (161)
Counter-irritants, embrocations, rubs	16% (80)	*	16% (86)
Mouth and throat preparations	7% (133)	13% (23)	8% (156)
Cough and lower respiratory preparations	48% (130)	29% (48)	43% (178)
Antacids, indigestion remedies	19% (202)	4% (27)	17% (229)
Sticking plasters, bandages, corn pads, dressings, poultices	12% (109)	*	13% (126)
Laxatives, health salts	10% (233)	0% (27)	9% (260)
Tonics	27% (22)	*	21% (29)
Iron, vitamin, mineral preparations	41% (175)	8% (48)	34% (223)
Slimming preparations	*	*	*
Other nutritional and metabolic preparations	80% (39)	*	81% (43)
Eye preparations	30% (53)	*	32% (59)
Ear preparations	*	*	*
Upper respiratory and nose preparations	24% (62)	*	27% (79)
Antihistamines, cold remedies	*	*	60% (20)
Sedatives, sleeping pills, tranquillisers	100% (152)	*	100% (158)
Antidepressants, stimulants	*	*	*
Antinauseants, travel sickness preparations	*	*	20% (20)
Other drugs acting on the CNS	*	*	*
Antibiotic, antiseptic, fungicidal, keratolytic ointments and powders	18% (74)	15% (27)	17% (101)
Barrier creams, insect repellent creams, suntan lotions	*	*	*
General antiseptics, germicides, disinfectants, cleaners	0% (65)	*	0% (78)
Corticosteroid skin preparations	96% (53)	*	94% (69)
Antirheumatic preparations, corticosteroids	95% (20)	*	95% (21)
Hormones	*	*	*
Contraceptive pills	100% (49)	*	100% (49)
Genito-urinary preparations	87% (30)	*	87% (30)
Suppositories, rectal preparations	*	*	*
Antidiarrhoea preparations	*	*	*
Cardio-vascular preparations	100% (45)	*	100% (45)
Antibiotics, anti-infective agents, anthelmintics	100% (34)	100% (25)	100% (59)
Ordinary food and drinks used medicinally (e.g. alcohol, honey)	0% (156)	*	1% (174)
Diet	*	*	*
Herbal remedies	*	*	*
Surgical clothing, trusses, appliances, elastic stockings	69% (65)	*	70% (67)
Not elsewhere classifiable	*	*	*
Unidentified	87% (330)	81% (36)	86% (366)
All medicines	36% (3,161)	26% (566)	35% (3,727)

* Less than twenty medicines.

The Nature of Medication

of the different types of medicine that were prescribed are shown in Table 16. Only a tenth of the analgesics, skin creams, laxatives and mouth and throat preparations used by adults were obtained on a prescription. The symptoms for which these common non-prescribed medicines were taken were also among the most frequently reported. As symptoms like sore throats, colds, coughs, headache, indigestion, rheumatism, and skin trouble are so common people become familiar with them. They are also symptoms for which there were reputed remedies before the advent of modern therapeutics, so the treatment of these symptoms by home medication is a long-standing part of our culture. Prescribed medicines, and the symptoms they were taken for, are less common and less familiar.

Relationship between self-medication and prescription

TABLE 17   A comparison of those who had and those who had not taken prescribed medicines showing the proportion who had taken non-prescribed medicines at different levels of symptom reporting

	Proportion who had taken non-prescribed medicines among adults who had:	
	taken prescribed medicines	not taken precribed medicines
Number of symptoms:		
None	a	12% (108)
One	46% (67)	52% (163)
Two	54% (81)	72% (152)
Three	60% (75)	75% (107)
Four	74% (62)	80% (108)
Five	76% (62)	90% (62)
Six	84% (45)	93% (45)
Seven	83% (40)	91% (33)
Eight or more	84% (136)	94% (51)
All adults	69% (582)	66% (829)

The figures in brackets are the bases from which percentages were calculated.

a There were only 12 people in this group; one had taken a non-prescribed medicine.

The Nature of Medication

Prescribed and non-prescribed medication are not of course mutually exclusive forms of behaviour. When people have symptoms they may take some self-prescribed medicines, get a prescription from the doctor, do both of these or neither. The taking of prescribed and non-prescribed medicines may be independent activities, alternatives or one may supplement the other. During the two weeks asked about in the survey 28% of the adults had taken at least one item of both kinds of medicine, 13% had taken only prescribed, 39% only self-prescribed medicines, and 20% none. This suggests at first sight that the two activities are independent: whether or not a person took self-prescribed medicines seemed unrelated to whether or not they took prescribed medicine. Sixty-nine per cent of those taking prescribed medicines had also taken self-prescribed ones, and a similar proportion, 66%, of those not taking prescribed medicine. But the more symptoms people had the more likely they were to do either of these, and when adults with the same number of symptoms are compared we find that those who had taken prescribed medicines were less likely to take self-prescribed ones than those who had not done so. This is shown in Table 17. These data suggest that self-medication is often used as an alternative to consulting the doctor.[5] Further evidence to support this comes from Table 18 which compares the estimated average number of general practitioner consultations for those who had taken none, one and two or more self-prescribed medicines.[6] At all levels of symptom reporting those adults who had taken two or more self-prescribed medicines had lower consultation rates than those taking one, and those taking one self-prescribed medicine had lower rates than

[5] This is contrary to the findings of Jefferys, Margot, Brotherston, J. H. F. and Cartwright, Ann, 1960, 'Consumption of medicines on a working-class housing estate'. In the present survey the findings on the relationship between self-medication and doctor consultation still held for working-class people alone. Possible reasons for the different findings are that the earlier study was confined to a single area, the proportion taking prescribed medicines was lower and the population covered was younger.

[6] The average number of consultations was estimated from answers to a question about whether they had had none, one, two to four, five to nine, or ten or more consultations in the previous twelve months. The measure is crude and is probably an under-estimate. The average was 3·6 for all adults whereas the estimate from the number of consultations in the previous two weeks was 5·2. Estimates from the last source show approximately similar but rather more erratic trends in the various analyses we have quoted.

31

those who had not taken any. At the same time the average number of consultations did not vary with the number of non-prescribed medicines they had taken when all the adults are considered together.[7] This apparent lack of relationship disappears when the

TABLE 18   *The relationship between non-prescribed medication, doctor consultation and number of symptoms for adults*

	Mean number of general practitioner consultations in the previous 12 months				
	Number of symptoms				*All adults*
Number of non-prescribed medicines taken in 2 weeks:	0 or 1	2 or 3	4 or 5	6 or more	
None	2·2 (221)	3·8 (137)	4·8 (59)	8·1 (45)	3·6 (463)
One	1·8 (102)	3·0 (145)	3·9 (83)	5·8 (81)	3·4 (411)
Two or more	1·3 (27)	2·6 (133)	3·1 (149)	5·1 (220)	3·7 (530)

The figures in brackets are the numbers for which means were calculated.

amount of illness, measured by the number of symptoms reported, is taken into account. Taking prescribed medicines was of course strongly related to professional consultation. The proportion of adults who had taken any prescribed medicine in the two weeks before interview rose from 9% of those who had not consulted their doctor at all in the previous year to 84% of those who had consulted ten or more times. What other differences were there between those people taking prescribed and non-prescribed medicines?

Some differences between those who had taken only non-prescribed, only prescribed and both kinds of medicine are shown in Table 19. The people who had used both kinds reported more symptoms and rated their health lower than other people taking only one kind. They had also taken more medicines. When those who had taken only prescribed medicines are compared with those who had taken only non-prescribed ones there is no difference between them in the number of medicines they had taken or in the number of symptoms they reported. But the type of symptom did vary. Those taking only non-prescribed medicines

[7] Similar findings are reported by Kalimo, E., 1969, *Determinants of Medical Care Utilization*, p. 29.

reported some symptoms more frequently than did those taking only prescribed medicines: headaches (49% compared with 21%), coughs, catarrh and phlegm (34% against 26%), indigestion (22% and 9%), sore throats (15% and 4%), cuts, burns and bruises (13% and 3%). Symptoms more prevalent among those taking

TABLE 19 *Some differences between adults who had taken only prescribed, only self-prescribed and some of each kind of medicine during a two-week period*

	All non-prescribed	All prescribed	Some of each
Proportion rated health:	%	%	%
Excellent or good	77	57	45
Fair or poor	23	43	55
Mean number of symptoms in previous two weeks	3·9	3·6	5·8
Mean number of general practitioner consultations in previous twelve months	1·9	6·8	6·0
Mean number of prescribed medicines taken in two weeks	—	2·0	1·9
Mean number of non-prescribed medicines taken in two weeks	2·0	—	2·2
Proportion aged 55 or more	32%	52%	44%
Number of adults (= 100%)[a]	549	182	399

[a] Small numbers for whom inadequate information was obtained have been omitted when calculating averages and percentages.

prescribed medicines only were muscle and joint pains (32% against 26%), sleeplessness (19% and 12%), swollen ankles (14% and 6%), palpitations (9% and 5%), faintness and dizziness (13% and 6%), and nerves, depression and irritability (24% and 17%). Those who had taken only prescribed medicines had more consultations and more often rated their health as fair or poor. They were also older and, as we showed earlier, the proportion taking prescribed medicines increased with age: but there was no variation in the proportion taking non-prescribed ones. Old people have rather more contact with their doctor than younger people although for women the distribution is U-shaped, the rate also being high during the child-bearing ages (see Table 20). Old people also suffer more often from chronic disorders and for some of these effective medicines are available only on prescription.

TABLE 20   *Consultation rates by age and sex: Average number of consultations during previous twelve months*

	Men	Women
Age: 21–24	3·2 (34)	5·7 (47)
25–34	2·2 (107)	4·8 (122)
35–44	2·5 (148)	3·5 (141)
45–54	3·0 (131)	3·4 (137)
55–64	3·0 (119)	4·0 (137)
65–74	3·0 (88)	4·5 (102)
75 or more	4·2 (33)	5·9 (51)
All age groups	2·9 (660)	4·2 (745)

Figures in brackets are the numbers of adults for which the means were calculated.

Most of the elderly too, depend on pensions as the primary source of income [8] so may not be able to afford non-prescribed medicines. The difference in cost to the person for prescribed and non-prescribed medicines is greater for pensioners than for other adults because they are exempt from prescription charges. Children too are exempt from these charges. What is the pattern of their consultations and medications?

Children: consultation and medication

The relationship between prescribed and non-prescribed medication is rather different for children. Table 21 shows that, like the adults, those who had taken both kinds of medicines tended to have more reported symptoms and to have their health rated as fair or poor by their parents. They also had taken twice as many items of medicine as children who had taken only prescribed or

[8] Townsend, P. and Wedderburn, Dorothy, 1965, *The Aged in the Welfare State*, p. 77.

TABLE 21 *Some differences between children who had taken only prescribed, only self-prescribed and some of each kind of medicine during a two-week period*

	All non-prescribed	All prescribed	Some of each
Proportion whose health was rated:	%	%	%
Excellent or good	84	57	52
Fair or poor	16	43	48
Number of children (= 100%)	185	40	62
Mean number of symptoms	2·0 (184)	1·6 (40)	3·4 (62)
Mean number of general practitioner consultations in previous twelve months	3·0 (171)	3·6 (37)	5·2 (60)
Mean number of prescribed medicines taken in two weeks	—	1·5 (40)	1·5 (61)
Mean number of non-prescribed medicines taken in two weeks	1·6 (185)	—	1·8 (62)

The figures in brackets are the numbers of children for which the means were calculated.

non-prescribed medicines. However, unlike the adults, those who had taken both kinds had had more consultations with general practitioners during the previous twelve months than the others. This suggests that parents of children with multiple symptoms tend to use self-medication and doctor consultation to supplement one another. This is borne out by the data presented in Table 22.

TABLE 22 *Variation in prescribed and non-prescribed medication with doctor consultation for children*

	Number of general practitioner consultations in the previous 12 months				
	0	1	2–4	5–9	10+
Proportion taking:					
Prescribed medicine	5%	15%	24%	44%	39%
Non-prescribed medicine	34%	42%	52%	63%	78%
Number of children (= 100%)	134	122	154	59	23

Not only does the proportion of children taking prescribed medicine increase with the rate of general practitioner consultation, but so does the proportion taking non-prescribed medicine. Thirty-four per cent of those children who had not seen their general practitioner during the past year had taken a non-prescribed medicine; this rose to 78% of those who had seen him ten or more times. Results from another study suggest that some mothers use different parts of the health service to supplement one another.[9] More mothers who consulted the general practitioner about children's colds were attending an infant welfare clinic than mothers who had not consulted. In addition, and again unlike the adults, those children who had taken a non-prescribed medicine had higher average rates of general practitioner consultation than those who had not taken any self-prescribed medicine. Table 23 shows this for two levels of symptom reporting.

TABLE 23   *The relationship between non-prescribed medication, doctor consultation and number of symptoms for children*

	Mean number of general practitioner consultations in the previous 12 months		
	Number of symptoms		All children
	0 and 1	2 or more	
No non-prescribed medicines taken	1·8 (225)	3·5 (36)	2·0 (261)
One or more non-prescribed medicines taken	2·5 (88)	4·2 (143)	3·6 (231)

The numbers in brackets are the numbers of children for whom the means were calculated.

Summary

Aspirins and other pain-killers were the medicines most commonly taken by adults; skin ointments and antiseptics by children. The majority of both of these were not prescribed. Most are palliatives, relieving the common symptoms of headaches, colds, rashes and

Waller, Jane, 1971, 'Some factors associated with use of medical services for a trivial condition'.

skin abrasions. Almost a fifth of the prescribed medicines were ones acting on the central nervous system.

For adults it was found that professional treatment and self-medication were sometimes alternatives. Although there was no correlation between medical consultations and the number of non-prescribed medicines taken when all adults were considered together, when the number of symptoms reported was held constant the two were negatively associated. For children the situation was different, medical consultation and self-treatment being positively correlated both for all children and at different sickness levels. For them self-treatment was apparently used to supplement professional consultation.

4

FREQUENCY AND LENGTH OF MEDICATION

How do prescribed and non-prescribed medicines compare with one another in the frequency with which they are used and the length of time over which they are taken? After answering this the chapter looks in detail at repeat prescribing and then, more briefly, at the under-use of prescribed medicines.

How often?

A fifth of the medicines taken by adults in the two weeks before they were interviewed had been taken only once during this time; two-fifths had been taken ten or more times.[1] Table 24 also shows that prescribed medicines were taken more often than non-prescribed ones. Sixty-nine per cent of the prescribed items had been taken ten or more times in the two weeks, 26% of the non-prescribed. This difference in the frequency with which they were used means that of the medicines taken in the last twenty-four hours a higher proportion, 49% were prescribed, compared with 36% in the last two weeks.

Aspirin and other pain-killers were the most commonly taken type of medicine, and generally these were not prescribed. Table 25 below shows that they were taken on average less frequently than most other medicines. More than a third of the analgesics had been taken only once during the two weeks before the interview. Fourteen per cent of them had been taken ten or more times, which is equivalent to nearly once a day, 8% were reported to be taken every day.[2] Laxatives were also taken relatively infrequently. The types of medicines taken relatively frequently were mainly those where a high proportion were prescribed such as

[1] 'How many times have you taken/used _____ in the last two weeks?'
[2] IF TAKEN IN LAST 24 HOURS 'Do you take/use it every day?'

preparations acting on the central nervous system and cardio-vascular, genito-urinary preparations and antibiotics. But tonics and vitamins were also taken regularly, and less than half of them were prescribed. Prescribed medicines may be taken

TABLE 24 *Frequency with which prescribed and non-prescribed medicines were taken by adults in two weeks before interview*

	Prescribed	Non-prescribed	All medicines
Number of times taken in two weeks before interview:	%	%	%
Once	6	26	19
Twice	5	17	13
3–4	8	17	14
5–9	12	14	13
10–24	38	21	24
25–39	15	3	10
40 or more	16	2	7
Estimated mean number of times taken	17	7	10
Proportion taken every day	62%	20%	35%
Number of medicines (= 100%)	1,133	1,975	3,108

regularly as a course of treatment with a specific dose to be taken at definite intervals. Non-prescribed ones, often used to relieve symptoms, are likely to be taken more irregularly. But people may self-prescribe a course of vitamins or tonics in an attempt to help a general feeling of malaise or in the hope that it will prevent illness. Three-quarters of the non-prescribed tonics and vitamins had been taken ten or more times during the two-week period.

Up to now we have described the frequency with which various medicines were taken. Looking at it instead from the point of view of people we find that two-fifths of the adults had taken an item of medicine at least once every day of the two weeks in question. Twenty-eight per cent had taken a prescribed medicine at least once daily, 20% had done so with a non-prescribed medicine. So medicine taking is not only a common but also a frequent activity for many people. How long do they go on taking the same sorts of medicines?

TABLE 25 Frequency with which different medicines were taken by adults

Pharmacological classification (grouped)[a]

Number of times taken in two weeks before interview	Analgesics and antipyretics (01)	Preparations acting on the C.N.S. (39, 30, 3X, 3Y)	Antacids and indigestion remedies (90)	Laxatives (08)	Tonics, iron, vitamins and minerals (19, 10)	Hormones and oral contraceptives (50, 5X)	Slimming and other nutritional and metabolic preparations (1X, 1Y)	Preparations acting on the respiratory system (50)	Preparations acting on the ear, nose and throat (04, 20, 2X)	Preparations acting on the skin (02, 49, 40, 4X, 4Y)	Eye Preparations (29)	Medicinal food and drink (79, 70, 7X)	Dressings and appliances (89, 07)	Cardio-vascular and genito-urinary preparations (6X, 5Y)	Preparations acting systemically on infections (6Y)	Preparations used in rheumatic diseases (03, 59)	Rectal and diarrhoea preparations and those for allergies (69, 60, 2Y)
	%	%	%	%	%	%	%	%	%	%	%	%	%	%	%	%	%
Once	34	7	22	34	3	4	2	9	15	17	15	18	20	4	6	16	20
Twice	26	5	16	16	3	—	4	10	5	13	19	9	11	1	3	21	13
3–4	16	7	23	18	8	7	2	14	18	19	11	11	7	5	12	16	20
5–9	10	11	9	11	6	24	8	22	20	18	23	18	9	15	3	13	13
10–24	10	43	17	20	45	65	47	22	30	27	26	38	52	28	42	22	25
25–39	3	12	4	1	16	—	16	8	7	5	4	1	1	27	21	8	8
40+	1	15	9	—	19	—	21	15	5	1	2	5	—	20	12	4	1
Estimated mean number of times	5	17	9	5	19	10	20	14	11	8	8	9	8	20	19	8	9
Proportion taken every day	8%	67%	20%	20%	67%	84%	77%	32%	25%	28%	26%	40%	53%	76%	41%	29%	23%
Number of medicines (= 100%)	620	179	198	229	192	54	49	129	199	291	53	165	168	74	33	98	40

How long?

Two-thirds of the items of medicine taken by adults were ones they had first tried at least a year before the interview.[3] Non-prescribed medicines were longer-standing remedies than prescribed ones; only a quarter had first been used within the previous year compared with half the prescribed items. This is shown in Table 26. More than half of the items of self-prescribed

TABLE 26   *Length of time since first used or had prescription for medicine*

	First used non-prescribed medicine	*First had prescription for prescribed medicine*
	%	%
Less than 2 weeks ago	8	13
2 weeks < 1 month	3	10
1 month < 6 months	7	16
6 months < 1 year	6	10
1 year < 5 years	21	31
5 years < 10 years	13	11
10 years or more	42	9
Number of medicines (= 100%)	1,948	1,116

analgesics and laxatives taken by adults were well-tried remedies that had first been used more than ten years before the interview. Nearly all the kinds of prescribed drugs taken by the adults followed the general pattern shown in Table 26 except the preparations acting on infections and immunological preparations, 64% of which had first been prescribed during the two weeks preceding the interview.

Repeat prescriptions

Since so many of the adults' prescribed medicines had been taken or used over long periods of time it is not surprising that nearly three-quarters of them were obtained on repeat prescriptions. An

[3] 'When did you first take/use _____?' or 'How long ago did you first get a prescription for _____?'

estimate of the proportion of prescriptions which were repeats comes from the sample of 399 prescriptions obtained in the two weeks before the interview.[4] Sixty-five per cent were for medicines the person had been given prescriptions for before. Another study specifically concerned with repeat prescribing found that 41% of doctors' contacts resulted in a repeat prescription.[5] In the present study a repeat prescription was given at 33% of the consultations that adults had had with their doctor during the two weeks before the interview. Balint and his colleagues also found that 62% of repeat prescription regimes were a year or more old. The comparable proportion in this study was 70%.

TABLE 27   *Number of prescriptions for same medicines*

Number of prescriptions:	%
One	29
Two	9
Three	7
Four	4
Five to nine	12
Ten to nineteen	12
Twenty to thirty-nine	9
Forty or more	18
Number of prescribed medicines taken in two weeks (= 100%)	1,086

People were not asked whether they had taken their prescribed medicines continuously since they were first prescribed them, but Table 27 shows that many of the prescriptions had been repeated several times.[6] For a fifth of the medicines, forty or more prescriptions had been written.

When more than one prescription had been obtained for the

[4] People who had consulted a doctor during this time were asked if he gave them a prescription or medicine and if so for how many things. In addition everyone was asked: 'In the last two weeks have you got a prescription either by phoning up, writing for it, getting a repeat from the doctor's receptionist or in any other way that did not involve seeing the doctor, or any prescription from the dentist?' and then: 'Were there any (other) prescriptions you were given in the last two weeks that you did not necessarily get made up or take?'
[5] Balint, Michael; Hunt, John; Joyce, Dick; Marinker, Marshall and Woodcock, Jasper, 1970. *Treatment or Diagnosis*, p. 7, and p. 19.
[6] 'How many prescriptions for _____ have you had altogether?'

same drug people were asked whether they usually saw the doctor or not when they got a repeat. For almost half, 48%, people said they always saw the doctor; 31% said they usually did not. A quarter of the prescriptions adults received in the two weeks before interview were obtained without seeing the doctor. The more frequently the same item had been prescribed the less likely the patient was to see the doctor. Fourteen per cent of repeats which had been previously prescribed four or less times were usually obtained without seeing the doctor. The proportion rose to 41% for items which had been prescribed twenty or more times. This substantiates Balint's finding[7] that repeat prescription patients often have 'indirect contacts' with their doctors.

The kinds of medicines that were most likely to be repeatedly prescribed were cardio-vascular and genito-urinary drugs: 63% had been repeated ten or more times. Between 35% and 48% of the digestive system remedies, analgesics, central nervous system drugs, nutritional, metabolic and hormonal preparations (not oral contraceptives) and skin medicaments taken or used had been obtained on the tenth or more repeat prescription for the same item. These groups of medicines made up most of those first prescribed a year or more before the interview. This can be seen from Table 28. An analysis of long-term (six months or more) repeat prescriptions written by a group of doctors also found that preparations acting on the central nervous system were the medicines most often prescribed in those circumstances.[8]

Three hundred and sixty-three (26%) of the adults in the study reported having taken at least one item of prescribed medicine that had first been prescribed a year or more before being interviewed. Sixty-six per cent of these people had taken only one item but 19% had taken two and the remaining 15% three or more, all of which had first been taken at least a year previously. Women were more likely than men to be taking medicines first prescribed a year or more ago: 31% compared with 20%. There was also a trend with age, increasing from 11% of those aged 21–24 to 55% of people aged 75 or more. Table 28 also shows that a third of the people taking medicines first prescribed at least a year earlier, that is 8% of all adults in the sample, were taking drugs acting on the central nervous system and had been doing so for a year or

7 Balint, Michael, *et al.*, op. cit., p. 46.
8 Balint, Michael, *et al.*, op. cit., p. 64.

TABLE 28 *The nature of long-term prescribing*

	Medicines first prescribed a year or more before interview	Proportion of people taking medicines first prescribed a year or more ago [b]
	%	%
Analgesics and antipyretics (01)	7	10
Preparations acting on the C.N.S. (39, 30, 3X, 3y)	24	32
Antacids and indigestion remedies (06)	6	7
Laxatives (08)	3	4
Tonics, iron, vitamins and minerals (19, 10)	6	9
Hormones and oral contraceptives (50, 5X)	7	11 [a]
Slimming and other nutritional and metabolic preparations (1X, 1y)	6	8
Preparations acting on the lower respiratory system (05)	6	7
Preparations acting on the ear, nose and throat (04, 20, 2X)	1	2
Preparations acting on the skin (02, 49, 40, 4X, 4y)	10	13
Eye preparations (29)	1	1
Dressings and appliances (89, 07)	8	12
Cardio-vascular and genito-urinary preparations (6X, 5y)	10	10
Preparations acting systemically on infections (6y)	1	1
Preparations used in rheumatic diseases (03, 59)	3	4
Rectal and diarrhoea preparations and those for allergies (69, 60, 2y)	1	3
Total number of long-term prescriptions and adults taking them (= 100%)	455	304

[a] The proportion is 1% if people taking oral contraceptives are excluded.
[b] Proportions add up to more than 100% because some patients had taken more than one type of medicine.

more, although we do not know if they had all done so continuously. Over half of this group, 56%, were taking more than one long-term prescribed medicine compared with 30% of those taking long-term drugs of other kinds only.

Central-nervous-system drugs were the type most commonly taken by those taking long-term prescribed medicines. Other medicines taken or used by a tenth or more of them were analgesics and anti-pyretics, hormones and oral contraceptives, preparations acting on the skin, cardio-vascular and genito-urinary preparations and dressing and appliances.

Joyce has suggested that any drug that has been taken for longer than two years has a large symbolic component on which patients may be psychologically dependent.[9] However there are patients, such as diabetics, on long-term drug therapy who should not be included in this category. But if we accept Joyce's contention then results from the study seem to substantiate his estimate that one in five of all prescriptions may be written by general practitioners for their symbolic functions and that there are between one and one and a half million patients in Great Britain dependent on the symbolic functions of prescribed drugs.

Medicines obtained on repeat prescription were thought to be more efficacious than those obtained for the first time. A subjective appraisal of the efficacy of all the medicines taken in the study was made by asking people whether each of the medicines they used helped 'a lot', 'some' or 'not at all'. Two-thirds of both the prescribed and non-prescribed medicines were thought to have helped the symptom they were taken for 'a lot'. However, overall, non-prescribed medicines were reported to be rather more effective than prescribed ones. Twenty-three per cent were felt to help to 'some' extent compared with 17% of prescribed medicines. People were uncertain about the efficacy of only 6% of non-prescribed items compared with 10% of the prescribed. And the proportions that had not helped at all were 4% of the non-prescribed, 5% of the prescribed ones. The proportion said to have helped 'a lot' increased from 56% of those on a first prescription to 78% of those prescribed ten or more times. Drugs that were thought not to be helpful tended not to be taken as often as advised. This is discussed in the next section.

[9] Joyce, C. R. B., 1969, 'Quantitative estimates of dependence on the symbolic function of drugs'.

Under-use?

Wilson and Enoch found a substantial amount of drug rejection in a study of patients in hospital where nurses handed out the tablets.[10] Bonnar *et al.* found that after two months 32% of a group of pregnant women attending an ante-natal clinic had stopped taking their iron.[11] What happens to drugs prescribed in general practice? Linnett has suggested that there is only a 50% chance of them being taken at all.[12] It is not possible to make a definite estimate of this from an interview survey with patients, but we tried to get some idea of the size of the problem.

The first question is whether or not the patient had the prescription made up. Seven per cent of the 399 prescriptions obtained in the last two weeks had not been made up at the time of interview, mainly because people had only just got the prescription or had not yet finished their present supply. Only two people had no intention of getting their prescriptions made up. One, a woman, had been prescribed four items but she did not get any of them made up:

> because the specialist advised me not to take anything. I don't really know why I went to the doctor because he gave me prescriptions for the same things and I'm not going to use them, but I didn't want to hurt his feelings so I took the prescription and said nothing.

The other was a man who said:

> I recently bought some—Ralgex—on advice from a friend. The doctor prescribed the same thing so I didn't get it.

Diary information, obtained for 73% of the prescriptions, showed that all but six (the five given to the two people quoted above and one other) of the prescriptions were made up and tried during the following two weeks. Of the prescriptions that had been made up at the time of interview 7% had not been tried. The diaries showed that all but three had been taken within the following two weeks. This suggests that on the whole people do

[10] Wilson, J. D. and Enoch, M. D., 1967, 'Estimation of drug rejection by schizophrenic in-patients with analysis of clinical factors'.
[11] Bonnar, J., Goldberg, A., Smith, J. A., 1969, 'Do pregnant women take their iron?'
[12] Linnett, M., 1968, 'Prescribing habits in general practice.'

bother to get their prescriptions made up and to try them. However diary information was not obtained about 12 of the prescriptions which had not been made up or tried. This means that the proportion of prescriptions not tried lies somewhere between 2% and 5%. Most of these would not be made up.[13] The next question is whether they took them as advised. People were asked whether they took their prescribed medicines more, less or exactly as they had been advised. They said they had not been advised how to take 4% of the medicines, but for the rest they said they took 80% of the medicines exactly as advised. Nineteen per cent were taken less than advised and rather fewer than 1% were taken more than advised. Over a third, 36%, of the medicines said not to help the symptom at all were taken less than advised. By far the most common reason given for not taking as much of a medicine as had been advised was that the person did not think it necessary to take it as often or in such large quantities as advised, that he only took it when he needed it or stopped when he was better. The next most commonly stated reason was that the person was to some extent 'anti-drugs', saying that he did not like taking drugs either at all, too often or too much or that he did not want to get into the habit. These two reasons seem to summarise many people's feelings towards medicines. On the one hand they can choose whether to take non-prescribed medicines or to go to the doctor for prescribed ones. They then feel free to a certain extent to decide when and how much to take. This freedom may lead in some cases either to taking the drugs in quantities insufficient for therapeutic effectiveness, or to continuing to take the drugs over long periods and developing a habit, getting their drugs on repeat prescriptions. On the other hand some people seem to be anxious about becoming dependent on a drug and about other more obscure dangers in taking potent medicines. This may be one of the reasons why self-medication is so popular.

[13] It is possible that being asked to keep a diary influenced people and made them more likely to take their medicines or get them made up. They did not of course know that only people who had been given a prescription were asked to keep diaries. Data from the pilot survey, when all the people interviewed were asked to keep diaries, showed similar proportions of people recorded taking medicines on a random day as reported doing so in the last twenty-four hours.

Children

Children's medicines were taken less frequently than adults' and, as expected, for a shorter time. Their prescribed medicines were less often repeats but even so the proportion was nearly half. The figures are in Table 29. A quarter of the children's medicines on repeat prescriptions were for antibiotics and other preparations acting systemically on infections. One in six were for preparations

TABLE 29   *The frequency and length of children's medication*

	Prescribed medicines	Non-prescribed medicines
Number of times taken in two-week period:	%	%
Once	12	37
Twice	7	20
3–4	12	13
5–9	16	11
10–24	32	17
25–39	11	1
40+	10	1
Mean number of times taken	14	5
Length of time since first taken:	%	%
Less than 2 weeks	28	16
2 weeks less than 1 month	19	3
1 month less than 6 months	16	10
6 months less than 1 year	9	14
1 year less than 5 years	27	38
5 years or more	1	19
Number of prescriptions:	%	
One	53	
Two	17	
Three	7	
Four	6	
5–9	4	
10–19	9	
20 or more	4	
Number of medicines (= 100%)[a]	146	399

[a] Small numbers for which inadequate information was available have been excluded when calculating percentages.

acting on the central nervous system, one in eight for skin preparations and a similar proportion for preparations acting on the ear, nose and throat.

Summary and conclusions

Many medicines are taken over long periods of time and two-fifths of the adults in the sample took some medicine every day in the two weeks before the interview. Prescribed medicines were taken more frequently than non-prescribed ones, and nearly three-quarters of them had been obtained on repeat prescriptions. A quarter of the adults were taking medicines first prescribed a year or more ago. So, for a sizeable proportion of people, medicine taking has become a habit often encouraged, or at least supported, by their doctors. Other researchers have interpreted the high rate of repeat prescribing as an indication of some inadequacy in the doctor–patient relationship.[14] In the next chapter we try to explore this possibility by looking at people's relationships with their doctors and seeing whether and how these are associated with their medicine-taking habits. Data from this study suggest that few prescribed medicines are not made up but a fifth were said to be used less than advised by the doctor.

[14] Balint, Michael, *et al.*, op. cit., p. 146.

WHO TAKES THE MEDICINES?

Most people take some medicines. Some adults rely mainly on prescribed medicines, others are more likely to use self-prescribed ones. Which they do depends partly on their symptoms. This chapter looks at some other variables which may help to explain their behaviour: social class, knowledge, their attitudes to the doctor, some aspects of their personality and, for children, their position in the family.

Social class [1]

There is disagreement at the present time about whether the middle class make better use of the National Health Service than the working class, or whether the system is working equitably.[2] To answer the question satisfactorily requires studies which take into account differential morbidity and need. Do the working-class people in this study have more symptoms than the others? Is their need greater? Table 30 shows that working-class people reported more symptoms for the previous two weeks and were more likely to regard their health as fair or poor than middle-class people. The working class also had more consultations with general practitioners during the previous twelve months. This suggests that the working class have a greater need for medical care and make more use of general practitioner services.[3]

When we compare people reporting similar numbers of symptoms we find that working-class people still consult their doctor more often than people in the middle classes (see Table 31).

Are there class differences in their medicine-taking behaviour?

[1] For a description of the classification of social class see Appendix VII.
[2] Titmuss, R. M., 1968, *Commitment to Welfare*; Rein, Martin, 1969, 'Social Class and the Health Service'; Alderson, M. R., 1970, 'Social class and the health service'.
[3] Age and social class did not appear to be related in this study.

TABLE 30 *Variations with social class in the number of symptoms reported and health rating of adults*

	Social class					
	I	II	III Skilled	III	IV	V
	Profes-sional	Inter-mediate	non-manual	Skilled manual	Semi-skilled	Un-skilled
Mean number of symptoms reported in 2-week period	3·4	3·7	3·6	4·0	4·0	4·6
Proportion who rated their health fair or poor	17%	28%	28%	36%	37%	43%
Estimated mean number of general practitioner consultations in 12 months	2·9	3·1	3·3	3·6	4·0	4·2
Number of adults[a] (= 100%)	65	260	186	514	218	82

[a] A small number for whom inadequate information was obtained have been excluded when the percentages and means were calculated.

TABLE 31 *Number of symptoms, social class and general practitioner consultation rate*

	Estimated mean number of general practitioner consultations in 12 months Number of symptoms						
	0	1	2	3	4	5	6+
Middle class: I, II and III non-manual	1·1 (43)	1·5 (94)	3·3 (92)	3·1 (61)	3·6 (66)	3·1 (51)	5·0 (104)
Working class: III manual, IV and V	1·8 (69)	2·6 (123)	2·8 (123)	3·5 (109)	3·7 (98)	3·8 (68)	5·7 (222)

The figures in brackets are the numbers of adults for which the means were calculated.

Table 32 shows that Social Class I had taken an average of 1·7 items during the two weeks, those in Social Class V 2·6. All the other classes had taken an average of 2·2 items. Similar differences are shown for prescribed and non-prescribed medicines separately. But all the differences are small and could have occurred by

TABLE 32   *Mean numbers of prescribed and non-prescribed medicines taken by adults in different social classes*

	Social class					
	I	II	III Skilled	III	IV	V
	Profes-sional	Inter-mediate	non-manual	Skilled manual	Semi-skilled	Un-skilled
Mean number prescribed medicines taken in 2 weeks	0·7	0·8	0·7	0·8	0·8	1·0
Mean number non-prescribed medicines taken in 2 weeks	1·1	1·4	1·5	1·4	1·4	1·6
Mean number of all medicines taken in 2 weeks	1·7	2·2	2·2	2·2	2·2	2·6
Number of adults for whom averages calculated (= 100%)	65	260	186	514	218	82

chance. The proportion of symptoms for which some medicine was taken did not vary systematically with social class, and the proportion of prescribed medicines obtained on repeat prescriptions was similar for working- and middle-class people. There were some differences in the proportions taking different kinds of medicines, the most notable being that middle-class people more often took sedatives than working-class people. This is discussed in more detail in Chapter 8.

Children of non-manual workers were reported as having an average of 1·6 symptoms each, manual workers' children 1·4. Sixty-three per cent of the non-manual workers' children had been given a medicine compared with 54% of the others. These differences are in the opposite direction to those for adults, but again they are small and could have occurred by chance. The general lack of social class differences in the extent of medicine use support the finding of another study[4] that 'social class was rarely of importance in explaining' differences. That study concluded that 'sound explanations . . . are not to be found in simple and readily available descriptive variables concerning social position, but are more likely to lie in the more complex areas of social interaction and role'. Other variables we considered were medical knowledge and reliance on the doctor. Both of these were related to social class.

Knowledge

Two questions can be interpreted as measuring knowledge to some extent. First, people were asked whether or not they thought five specified illnesses were catching.[5] A third of the adults gave five correct answers; another third, four; a fifth, three; and a tenth, two or less. About nine-tenths of people gave the correct answer for anaemia and diabetes—that they were not catching. Three quarters gave the right answer for bronchitis and tuberculosis. Only just over half thought that polio was catching. Other studies[6] have shown that socio-economic status is related to accurate knowledge about health and illness. Not surprisingly in this survey working-class people were less knowledgeable than the middle-class. Eighty-two per cent of people in Social Class I gave four or five correct answers. The proportion fell to 53% of people in Social Class V.

The second question possibly related to knowledge was: 'Do you agree, disagree or feel neutral about the following statement: "Making sure your bowels open every day is important for keeping healthy" ?'[7] Seventy-seven per cent of the adults agreed about the

[4] Wadsworth, M. E. J., Butterfield, W. J. H. and Blaney, R., 1971, *Health and Sickness: the Choice of Treatment*, p. 81.

[5] 'Which of these illnesses do you think it is possible to catch from someone else: diabetes, polio, bronchitis, T.B., anaemia?'

[6] Glasser, M. A., 1958, 'A study of the public's acceptance of the Salk vaccine program'.
Samora, J., Saunders, L. and Larson, R. F., 1961, 'Medical vocabulary knowledge among hospital patients', and 1962, 'Knowledge about specific diseases in four selected samples'.

[7] Connell, *et al.*, found that a range between three bowel actions weekly and three daily could be regarded as normal and the need for a universal daily bowel movement was a myth. See Connell, A. M., Hilton, C., Irvine, G., Lennard-Jones, J. E. and Misiewicz, J. J., 1965, 'Variation of bowel habit in two population samples'.

need for a daily bowel movement. The proportion who disagreed increased from 8% of those who gave correct answers to none or one of the other knowledge questions to 20% of those who got all five right. Again middle-class people were more likely to give the 'correct' answer than the working-class. Just over a

TABLE 33   *Social class differences in response to two questions possibly related to knowledge*

	Social class					
	I	II	III	III	IV	V
			Skilled			
	Profes-sional	Inter-mediate	non-manual	Skilled manual	Semi-skilled	Un-skilled
Proportion of people who gave 4 or 5 right answers to whether or not 5 conditions are catching	82%	75%	69%	68%	61%	53%
Proportion of people who disagreed that a daily bowel movement is important for keeping healthy	37%	20%	19%	14%	10%	7%
Number of adults (= 100%)ᵃ	65	260	186	514	218	82

ᵃ Small numbers for whom inadequate information was obtained have been excluded when calculating percentages.

third of those in Social Class I disagreed that a daily bowel movement was important. This proportion fell to less than a tenth of those in Social Class V. Details of these trends are shown in Table 33. However these differences in people's knowledge were not related to their medicine taking. Similar proportions of people who gave different answers to these questions had taken prescribed and non-prescribed medicines. And belief in the desirability of a daily bowel movement was surprisingly, unrelated to laxative taking.

Reliance on the doctor

We asked people to try to imagine what they would do in six illness situations: consult the doctor, treat themselves, do something else or nothing at all. The six situations that people were asked about to assess their reliance on the doctor are given in Table 34 which also shows the proportions of people who thought they would do different things. About three-quarters of the adults thought they would consult the doctor for a 'constant

TABLE 34 *Adults' predicted action for six conditions*

Proportion who would:	A constant feeling of depression for about three weeks	Difficulty in sleeping for about a week	A heavy cold with a temperature and running nose	A headache more than once a week for a month	A very sore throat for three days and no other symptoms	A boil that doesn't clear up in a week
	%	%	%	%	%	%
Consult the doctor	72	53	27	57	42	76
Do something themselves	7	17	62	29	45	17
Do nothing	12	25	7	9	9	4
Other	7	3	1	2	1	1
Do more than one	2	2	3	3	3	2
Number of adults (= 100%)[a]	1,412					

[a] Small numbers for whom inadequate information was obtained have been excluded when calculating percentages.

feeling of depression for about three weeks' and for 'a boil that doesn't clear up in a week'. The condition which was most likely to be ignored was the sleeplessness. A quarter of the adults thought they would do nothing if they had difficulty sleeping for a week.

Fewer middle-class people than working class gave answers which indicated reliance on the doctor. A third of those in Social Class I said they would consult the doctor about four or more of the conditions. This proportion rose to half of those in Social Class V. Another possible indicator of people's reliance on their doctor was a question, 'If you were worried about a personal problem that wasn't strictly a medical one, do you think you might discuss it with your doctor?' This too was related to social class. Almost half (46%) of the working class thought they would discuss a personal problem with their doctor, a third of the middle class.

Adults who said they would consult their doctor in five or six of the hypothetical situations were in fact more likely to have consulted a doctor in the two weeks before they were interviewed: 22% of them had done so compared with 14% of the others. The more situations they said they were likely to consult about the more likely they were to have taken a prescribed medicine. The proportion who had done so increased from 20% of those who said they would not consult the doctor in any of the six situations to 62% of those who would seek his advice about all of them. And people who said they would consult their doctor about a personal problem were more likely than the others to have taken a prescribed medicine during the two-week period: 46% compared with 38%. Reliance on the doctor was unrelated to self-medication.

People with several symptoms were no more likely than those with few to say they would consult their doctor in different situations. So ill health did not appear to make people more reliant on their doctor even though those who had consulted their doctor several times in the previous year were more likely to say they would consult him in the hypothetical situations. The proportion who said they would consult about four or more rose from 35% of those with no consultations in the previous year to 52% with five or more. This suggests that at all levels of sickness there are some people who are more dependent on the doctor and therefore more likely to take prescribed medicines than others.

Parents interviewed about children were asked rather similar questions about situations in which they would consult the doctor.[8] Responses are shown in Table 35. The majority, three-quarters or more, said they would consult the doctor in each of

[8] 'I have a list of conditions or symptoms which I will read to you. I would like you to try and imagine what you would do if your children had them. Would you consult the doctor, do something yourself or what would you do—or wouldn't you do anything?'

the four circumstances. The association between consultation rates and 'reliance on the doctor' was less strong for children than for adults, possibly because the situations we asked about did not differentiate between parents so much. Forty-seven per cent of parents of children who had not seen the doctor in the previous

TABLE 35　*The action parents thought they would take if their children were in four illness situations*

	Frequently recurring colds	*A child who still wet the bed when he was five*	*A rash you were fairly certain was chicken pox when a lot of other children had it*	*A sore throat for three days and no other symptoms*
Proportion whose parents would:	%	%	%	%
Consult the doctor	82	83	93	76
Do something themselves	13	4	6	17
Do nothing	2	10	—	3
Other	1	2	—	1
Do more than one	2	1	1	3
Number of children (= 100%)ᵃ		519		

ᵃ Small numbers of adults for whom inadequate information was obtained have been excluded when calculating percentages.

year said they would consult the doctor in all four situations, 58% of those whose children had seen the doctor. But the children's medicine-taking patterns did not seem to be related to their parents' reliance on the doctor for children's illnesses.

Self-reliance

In the same way that 'reliance on the doctor' was related to prescribed medication, reliance on self-treatment was associated with self-medication. Adults who had not taken any self-prescribed medicine in the last two weeks said they would self-treat an average of 1·6 of the situations (listed in Table 34), and this average rose to 2·3 for those who had taken five or more self-prescribed medicines. Affirmative answers to two other questions suggest a degree of independence in health matters. People were asked whether they agreed or disagreed with the statement 'a person understands his own health better than most doctors do'. A quarter of the adults agreed with this. These 'independent' people reported more symptoms than the others, an average of 4·2 compared with 3·6. Even so, they were less likely to have consulted their doctor during the previous year than those who disagreed, 68% compared with 74%. They did not differ however in the medicines they had taken.

Adults were also asked which of two kinds of people they thought most like themselves: 'Doctors don't know everything about you so I don't always do exactly what they advise' or 'I always try to do exactly what the doctor advises even if it is not very pleasant or easy'. The majority, 86%, felt they were most like the second person. But this too was unrelated to their medicine taking. It was however linked with their views on the efficacy of the prescribed medicines they had taken. Of the prescribed medicines taken by people who thought they were most like the person who would not always do what the doctor advised, 46% were rated as having helped 'a lot', compared with 68% of those taken by people who thought they were most like the example of a person who tried to do exactly what the doctor said. People may have felt more sceptical about doctors' instructions because they were at the time of the interview taking an item of medicine that was not particularly effective. However this relationship demonstrates the way in which people's attitudes towards medical care may contribute to the efficacy of a drug. Self-reliant people, who felt 'a person understands his own health better than most doctors do', had lower expectations about doctors' ability to cure or relieve various conditions. They had less faith in doctors.

Faith in doctors

People were asked whether they thought doctors could cure completely, relieve or do very little about nine conditions or symptoms.[9] The conditions or symptoms are listed in Table 36 together with the replies. People were least optimistic about the ability of doctors to cure rheumatism and arthritis—less than one in twenty expected them to do this. But almost a quarter thought they could cure bronchitis and a similar proportion expected

TABLE 36   *Faith in doctors*

Thinks doctors can generally:	*Rheumatism*	*A bad cold*	*Corns*	*Skin cancer*	*Arthritis*	*Depression*	*Sleeplessness*	*Frequent headaches*	*Bronchitis*
	%	%	%	%	%	%	%	%	%
Cure	1	22	36	23	3	25	29	29	24
Help	78	50	27	36	75	59	63	58	68
Not help	14	26	15	7	16	11	4	5	3
Don't know/uncertain	7	2	22	34	6	5	4	8	5
Number of adults (= 100%)[a]	1,412								

[a] Small numbers of adults for whom inadequate information was obtained have been excluded when calculating percentages.

them to cure a bad cold. On the other hand another quarter thought doctors could do nothing for a bad cold and about a sixth felt they could not help to relieve arthritis and rheumatism. A tenth thought this about depression. Faith in doctors' ability to cure or relieve one condition was associated with a belief in their skill to help with others. For example 83% of those who felt he could cure or relieve a bad cold thought he could do one of these things for arthritis, compared with 66% of those who did not think he could help a cold.

The proportion who felt 'a person understands his own health better than most doctors' fell from a third of those with low expectations or faith in doctors to a fifth of those with high expectations.[10] But faith in doctors' ability to cure and relieve conditions did not seem to be related to frequency of consultation

[9] 'There are some things that doctors can cure completely, others that they can make feel better and some that they can do very little about. Do you think they can generally cure, help or not help: rheumatism', etc.
[10] Answers to the questions about whether doctors could cure or relieve different conditions were summarised by scoring two for conditions they thought doctors could cure and one for conditions he could relieve. Details are in Appendix V.

or to taking medicines. Possibly our measure of this attribute was too crude and confused with other factors like knowledge, although it did not in fact correlate with our knowledge score.

Personality differences

We looked at measures of two personality dimensions: extra-version–introversion and neuroticism–stability, each scored on a seven-point scale devised by S. B. G. and H. J. Eysenck.[11] At first it appeared that those with a high neuroticism score took more medicines than those with a low score on this scale: those with a score of four or more had taken an average of 2·9 medicines, those with a lower score an average of 2·1. But neuroticism was strongly linked with symptom reporting. People with a score of none reported an average of 2·5 symptoms each. This rose to an average of 6·1 reported by those with scores of five or six on the neuroticism scale. When the number of symptoms was held constant there was no association between neuroticism and the average number of medicines taken but there was some sugges-tion that those with a high score were more likely to have taken prescribed medicines and they seemed to consult their doctors more often. This is shown in Table 37.

TABLE 37   *The relationship between neuroticism score, the number of reported symptoms and consultation and prescribed medicine taking*

	Number of symptoms			
	0 or 1	2 or 3	4 or 5	6 or more
	Mean number of consultations in twelve months			
Neuroticism—low[a]	1·8 (272)	2·8 (275)	3·2 (182)	5·5 (150)
—high	2·9 (72)	3·7 (135)	4·6 (105)	5·8 (190)
	Proportion of adults who had taken prescribed medicine in last two weeks:			
Neuroticism—low	22% (258)	35% (276)	37% (183)	65% (152)
—high	26% (86)	42% (135)	50% (105)	61% (192)

[a] Low = score of 0, 1 or 2; high = score of 3, 4, 5, 6.
Figures in brackets are the numbers of adults for whom means and percentages were calculated.

---

[11] Further details are in Appendix V.

How much people talked about health was also related to neuroticism.[12] Three per cent said they did so a great deal, 13% fairly often, 67% only occasionally and 17% never. The average neuroticism score rose from 1·7 for those who never discussed it to 3·0 for those who said they talked about health and illness a great deal. Talking about health was also related to symptom reporting and to medicine taking in the same way as neuroticism. But of course these associations do not tell us whether people with high neuroticism scores perceive more symptoms, talk about their health and consult their doctors more often because they are 'neurotic' or whether ill health leads to neurosis and preoccupation with and discussion of illness. Extraversion–introversion did not seem to be related to ill health, consultation or medication.

First and only children

One variable we looked at for children was their position in the family. Douglas and Blomfield found that first-born children were most often taken to welfare centres and made more growth progress in their childhood.[13]

In the present study first and only children[14] were, on average, older than the others so it was necessary to control for age. Table 38 shows that at all ages first children were more often given some medicine than second children and, except for those aged 10–14, second children were more often given medicine than third or later ones. But in spite of being older—and older children had fewer symptoms than younger children—more symptoms were reported for first children than for others. The average number was 1·7 for first children, 1·4 for second and 0·9 for third or later ones. Once again differences in medication appear to be a reflection of perceived ill health.

[12] 'Do you talk about health and illness with your family and friends a great deal, fairly often, only occasionally or never?'
[13] Douglas, J. W. B. and Blomfield, J. M., 1958, *Children under Five*, p. 93 and also pp. 58–62 and 99.
[14] As the sample was confined to children under fifteen it is likely that some of the children who appear to be first born or only children in fact are not. This means that the effect of the position in the family is likely to be underestimated from these data.

TABLE 38   *The relationship between children's position in the family, age and the percentage who had been given medicine during a two-week period*

| | Proportion who had taken medicine | | |
| | Position of child in family | | |
	First	Second	Third or later
Age:			
Under 2 years	85% (27)	83% (24)	59% (17)
2 but less than 5	72% (53)	59% (29)	58% (31)
5 but less than 10	57% (61)	55% (62)	30% (46)
10 but less than 15	48% (116)	40% (40)	46% (13)
All ages	59% (257)	56% (155)	45% (107)
Mean number of medicines taken	1·2	1·1	0·7

Figures in brackets are the numbers of children on which the percentages were based (= 100%).

Discussion

Our attempt to identify medicine takers by such characteristics as age, sex and social class has been in many ways abortive. Apparent associations between age, social class and medication can be explained simply in terms of the amount of perceived ill health.

But the proportion taking medicines for their symptoms was related to some of their attitudes to, and relationships with, doctors. Those who were more likely to seek medical advice for particular conditions or to turn to their doctor when they had a personal problem, more often took medicines for their symptoms. Belief in doctors' ability to cure or relieve a number of conditions was not however related to their medicine-taking behaviour; neither was their medical knowledge. It might be expected that 'neurotic' people would want or need to rely more on medical help for advice and that this association would explain the observed relationship between neuroticism and medication. In fact neuroticism and our index of reliance on the doctor were unrelated. But neurotic people had more symptoms than others and even when this is taken into account they still consulted their doctor more often in practice although they did not predict they would do so when asked about hypothetical situations.

Whether or not people take medicines and consult their doctor in different situations seems to depend on many types of variables. We have been able to pin-point a few.

6

GENERAL PRACTITIONERS' VIEWS AND PRACTICES

So far we have looked at ill-health, consultation and medication from the point of view of patients. This chapter presents the attitudes and habits of their general practitioners. Many general practitioner consultations are probably initiated by patients.[1] What do doctors feel about the way they do this?

Appropriateness of consultations

In an earlier study a quarter of the general practitioners surveyed felt that half or more of their surgery consultations were for trivial, unnecessary or inappropriate reasons.[2] In the present survey doctors were asked what proportion, if any, of their consultations they would estimate were for ailments that people could treat or cope with themselves without seeing the doctor. Replies are shown in Table 39. A fifth of the doctors felt half or more consultations fell into that category, and half of the doctors thought it was at least a quarter. At the same time evidence is accumulating from a number of sources that many people, particularly among the elderly, do not consult their doctor about disabling conditions which he might be able to relieve.[3] So the expectations and actions of patients and doctors fail to match in two ways. The two sorts of discrepancy are illustrated in Table 40 which compares the proportion of doctors who thought various

[1] Cartwright, Ann, 1967, Unpublished data from *Patients and their Doctors*. Forty per cent of consultations reported by adults were felt to have been initiated by the doctor, for 48% it had been their own idea and for the remaining 12% a relative or other person had suggested it.

[2] Cartwright, Ann, 1967, op. cit., p. 44.

[3] Williamson, J., 1967, 'Detecting disease in clinical geriatrics', Lance, Hilary, 1971, 'Transport services in general practice', Cartwright, Ann; Hockey, Lisbeth and Anderson, J. L., *Life before Death* (in press).

TABLE 39 *Proportion of consultations felt to be for ailments people could treat or cope with themselves without seeing a doctor*

Proportion of consultations doctors feel are for ailments people could treat or cope with themselves	%
90% or more	—
75% but less than 90%	4
50% but less than 75%	16
25% but less than 50%	30
10% but less than 25%	34
5% but less than 10%	11
Less than 5%	5
Total number of doctors (= 100%)	322

TABLE 40 *Comparison of doctors' and adults' views on self-treatment in various circumstances*

	A constant feeling of depression for about three weeks	Difficulty in sleeping for about a week	A heavy cold with a temperature and running nose	A headache more than once a week for a month	A very sore throat for three days and no other symptoms	A boil that doesn't clear up in a week
Proportion of doctors who thought each condition suitable for people to treat themselves without consulting a doctor	9%	58%	86%	17%	27%	12%
Number of doctors (= 100%)	307					
Proportion of adults who thought they would do something themselves (including nothing) without consulting a doctor	26%	45%	70%	40%	55%	22%
Number of adults (= 100%)[a]	1,412					

[a] Small numbers of adults for whom inadequate information was obtained have been excluded when calculating percentages.

conditions suitable for people to treat themselves without consulting a doctor[4] with the proportion of adults who thought they would not consult a doctor about the same conditions. If we accept these predictions and views at their face value it seems that adults often may not consult doctors about depression, persistent headaches, acute sore throats and boils when doctors would feel this appropriate. On the other hand they may consult about sleeplessness and heavy colds more often than doctors feel reasonable.

The other main point that emerges from the data in Table 40 is the lack of unanimity among doctors. If doctors had exactly the same views on which of these conditions were suitable for self-treatment the proportions replying that each condition was suitable would be either 100% or 0%, and not the varying percentages shown in the table. As doctors are not unanimous about what conditions are appropriate for self-treatment it is not surprising that the variation in what patients think they would do is even greater. Nevertheless there was a correlation (+0·83) between the proportion of doctors and the proportion of patients who thought self-treatment appropriate for the various conditions. But patients cannot always foresee whether doctors will feel it is appropriate to be consulted about certain things. If they miscalculate and then feel rebuffed they may be less likely to consult in other circumstances which the doctor might be more sympathetic towards. In the earlier study of patients and their doctors it was found that the annual consultation rate of patients whose doctors considered few of their consultations to be for trivial reasons was higher than the rate of those patients whose doctors considered that many of their consultations were trivial.[5]

Results from this present study seem to substantiate the hypothesis based on these earlier findings that when a doctor regards a consultation as trivial, some patients are somehow discouraged from going to see him again. Table 41 shows that people whose general practitioners thought a high proportion of their consulta-

---

[4] 'Which of the following ailments do you think are generally suitable for most adults to treat themselves without consulting a doctor? (*a*) A constant feeling of depression for about three weeks, (*b*) Difficulty in sleeping for about a week, (*c*) A heavy cold with a temperature and running nose, (*d*) A headache more than once a week for a month, (*e*) A very sore throat for three days and no other symptoms, (*f*) a boil that does not clear up in a week'.

[5] Cartwright, Ann, 1967, op. cit., p. 51.

tions were for ailments that could be self-treated consulted him on average slightly less frequently than those whose doctors felt that only a small proportion fell into this category. This lack of agreement and understanding between patients and doctors may lead to different sorts of misapprehensions on other occasions, when people may be reluctant to 'bother the doctor' about conditions for which his help is more definitely needed.

TABLE 41   *Frequency of patient consultation and doctors' estimates of the proportion of their consultations which were for ailments that could be self-treated*

| | Proportion of consultations estimated by the general practitioner to be for ailments that could be self-treated | | | | |
	Less than 5%	5% < 10%	10% < 25%	25% < 50%	50% or more
Proportion of adults who had consulted their general practitioner five or more times during the past year	33%	24%	24%	22%	18%
Estimated annual consultation rate	4·5	4·0	3·6	3·7	3·2
Number of adults (= 100%)[a]	36	95	253	207	152

[a] This analysis is based on adults whose doctor participated in the study.

As most general practitioners estimated that at least a tenth of their consultations were for ailments people could treat or cope with themselves without seeing the doctor, we asked them if they thought anything should be done to try and reduce the number of consultations which patients make for minor ailments which are self-limiting and can be self-treated. A tenth of the general practitioners replied that nothing should be done to reduce the number of consultations for minor ailments. The most frequent suggestion made by the others was health education. Fifteen per cent suggested that education of patients by their own general practitioner was needed, 33% suggested general health education by local authorities and other bodies. These educational means were more often mentioned than financial disincentives, some form of which was suggested by a quarter of the doctors. A tenth of the doctors recommended the use of nursing staff to screen patients before they saw the doctor.

Self-treatment

Obviously many doctors regard self-treatment as appropriate for a substantial amount of illness. Do they do anything to encourage this among their patients? Nearly four-fifths (78%) of the doctors said they did something to encourage appropriate self-treatment among their patients, 73% said they tried to discourage inappropriate self-treatment.[6] Much of the encouragement consisted of telling patients that there was little the doctor could do for many minor ailments and anyway they were self-limiting. One doctor said:

I tell the patient they can treat most colds and chills as well or better than I can.

Doctors stressed the ineffectiveness of many medicines and several encouraged their patients to treat upper respiratory infections with aspirin. Others discouraged the use of that particular analgesic because of the irritating effect it has on the stomach.

Much of the general practitioners' advice to patients involved such forms of self-treatment as weight reduction and giving up smoking. One of the dangers of self-medication can be that it masks symptoms of serious disease. Many doctors said they talked to patients about this and tried to teach them which symptoms they should take straight to the doctor. The impression is not so much that doctors encourage and discourage self-medication but that they educate their patients about when and how to treat themselves and when and what to consult about. This service to patients is acknowledged by the adults in the study, nearly half of whom said they had learned something about the treatment of illness from their general practitioner.[7] A fifth said

[6] 'Do you do anything to encourage appropriate self-treatment among your patients?' 'Do you do anything to discourage inappropriate self-treatment among your patients?'
[7] 'I am going to read a short list of people and things which may influence peoples' knowledge about treatment of illness. Will you tell me whether you think you have learnt anything about treatment of illness from: television, your parents, other

that their doctors had been the most important source of this knowledge.

'He just answers questions straight—like putting my mind at ease over the pill. He tells me anything I want to know about the children.'

'My doctor has always had time to explain any illness or necessary remedy. He assumes you have the intelligence to understand and gives you the feeling that he is interested as well.'

'My doctor—he is very careful to explain and has explained a great deal to me about the change of life and how these pills will help me and I stick to taking them fourteen days before my period is due.'

'He tells us to cut down on cigarettes because it's no good for bronchitis and affects your heart probably and makes you breathless.'

'He tells you what to do, how to look after yourself, what precautions to take.'

More than half (58%) of the general practitioners said that during the two weeks before completing the questionnaire they had suggested that a patient should buy a medicine from a chemist without a prescription. A quarter said they had done so five or more times. So some doctors seem to do this fairly frequently, others not at all. Analgesics were the type of medicine most often recommended (by 37% of doctors) followed by local preparations for the skin, scalp and hair (by 20%). Remedies for the respiratory and digestive systems were each recommended by 17%. Thus the majority of doctors actively encouraged their patients to treat some of their own minor ailments and many of them suggested that they buy some of their own medicines from a chemist. There are other para-medical personnel such as pharmacists and local authority nurses who could give the public similar advice. What do general practitioners feel about them doing so? They were

---

relatives, your general practitioner, other doctors, radio, friends or neighbours, newspapers, magazines, books, health visitors or other nurses anywhere or anyone else (specify).

(*a*) 'Which of those do you think has been most helpful?'

(*b*) 'Can you give me some idea of the things you have learnt from them?'

asked whether the general public should be encouraged to ask health visitors, other nurses and pharmacists questions about health and medicines. Seventy-eight per cent of the doctors thought people should be encouraged to ask nurses, but they were much less enthusiastic about pharmacists. Thirty-one per cent of the doctors thought the public ought to be encouraged to ask pharmacists about health and medicines. This substantial minority shared the view of a general practitioner who did a small study on the public's use of pharmacists in eight English towns and concluded that 'the service given by the pharmacist to the public is valuable and one which saves the general practitioner a considerable amount of work'.[8]

Prescribing

At most consultations general practitioners give patients a prescription. Adults said they had done so at two-thirds of their consultations in the two-week study period.[9] This finding was included in the questionnaire we sent to the general practitioners. We asked them whether they thought they personally gave prescriptions more or less often than this or about as frequently.[10] Their replies suggest they thought this proportion might be an underestimate or that they wrote prescriptions more often than other doctors. Half of them thought they gave prescriptions at about two-thirds of their consultations but nearly half thought they gave one at more. Only 3% of the doctors estimated that they gave prescriptions at less than two-thirds of their consultations. Doctors may over-estimate the frequency with which they prescribe because of feelings of guilt about their prescribing habits. When they were asked: 'If you had more time to spend with each patient do you think you would give: fewer prescriptions, more prescriptions or the same number?' nearly half the doctors did not think the frequency of their prescribing would change, but more than half of them, 52%, thought they would write fewer prescriptions. Only 1% thought they would write

8 Whitfield, M., 1968, 'The pharmacists' contribution to medical care'.
9 This proportion was three-fifths of the children's consultations.
10 'At two-thirds of the consultations reported on our study patients said they had been given a prescription. Do you think you give prescriptions: at more consultations than this, at fewer, or at about the same proportion?'

more. The way more time with patients might cut prescribing is suggested by one doctor who said:

What people really want is to be listened to. Prescribing is rarely needed.

Doctors were also asked whether their prescribing would change in other ways if they had more time. Over half of them did not think so. A quarter of them thought they would prescribe in smaller quantities, a tenth thought the types of drugs they prescribed might change. Altogether 69% of doctors felt that their prescribing habits would be likely to change if they had more time to spend with patients.

To find out what doctors saw as the main factors influencing prescribing rates we asked them what they thought was the main reason for the variations in prescribing levels from one part of the country to another: different levels of sickness, different habits and attitudes of patients, different prescribing practices of general practitioners or something else. The different habits and attitudes of patients and the different prescribing practices of general practitioners were the most frequently perceived influences; the first was mentioned by nearly three-quarters of the doctors the second by over half. (Many doctors gave more than one answer.) Over a third mentioned different levels of sickness.

What are doctors' main sources of information about new drugs put on the market? Their replies to questions about this are shown in Table 42. Medical journals and drug-firm literature, representatives or meetings were most commonly cited as being the most helpful sources. The part played by the drug firms is further emphasised by the fact that nearly half the doctors, 45%, said they had seen five or more drug-firm representatives in the last four weeks. Only 6% had not seen any. But seeing representatives and relying on sources associated with the pharmaceutical industry for information did not seem to be related to their frequency of prescription nor to the cost of their prescribing. The Department of Health and Social Security provided three measures of the doctors' prescribing: average number of prescriptions per person on the doctor's list, average cost per prescription and average cost per person on the doctor's list. The doctors were given a score for each of the three measures. These scores relate to the average values for doctors whose prescribing was assessed during the same month of the year.[11]

While many doctors seem to feel that they prescribe too often and yet over-estimate the frequency with which they prescribe, they apparently under-estimate the proportion of prescriptions

TABLE 42   *General practitioners' sources of information about new drugs*

	Helpful source	Most helpful source
	%	%
Medical journals	82	25
Drug-firm literature, representatives or meetings	90	25
Monthly Index of Medical Specialities	68	14
British National Formulary	38	—
Prescribers' Journal	60	8
Letters from hospital consultants	65	11
Discussion with other doctors	57	7
Local clinical meetings	50	3
Refresher courses	71	7
Other sources	3	1
Number of doctors (= 100%)	325	298

obtained without seeing the doctor. They were asked whether the proportion of prescriptions they signed without seeing the patient was more or less than a fifth.[12] Forty-one per cent thought it was about the same proportion; more, 47%, thought it to be less and only 12% thought it more. Nearly all the doctors, 97%, had some arrangement whereby patients could obtain repeats without seeing the doctor. Only 3% of them would not sign prescriptions in the patient's absence.

The kinds of drugs which doctors thought they most frequently gave by repeat prescriptions without seeing patients[13] were sleeping tablets, tranquillisers and antidepressives. Three-fifths

[11] Further details about these scores are in Appendix II.
[12] 'One-fifth of the prescriptions the people on our study had had during a two-week period had been obtained without seeing the doctor. Do you think the proportion of prescriptions you sign without seeing the patient is more, less or about the same as this?'
[13] 'Which drugs, if any, are most commonly obtained on repeat prescriptions by your patients without seeing you?'

of the doctors mentioned these as some of the drugs most commonly obtained on repeat prescriptions. Nearly a half mentioned cardio-vascular and diuretic preparations. A third mentioned analgesics and similar preparations, nutritional preparations and respiratory system remedies. A quarter reported digestive system remedies, a fifth other drugs acting on the central nervous system and a tenth skin preparations. These compare reasonably well with the medicines reported by patients to have been obtained on a repeat prescription (see Table 28) and with data from a study of doctors' prescribing.[14]

Are there any drugs at present obtainable only on prescription that doctors would like to see freely available to the public?[15] Nine per cent of doctors thought there were. Some they mentioned were oral contraceptives, antihistamines, antibiotics and sulphonamides. More doctors, 25%, would like to restrict some drugs at present freely available.[16] Ten per cent thought more analgesics should be available only on prescription. Other suggestions were antihistamine cold cures, respiratory preparations for inhaling and some tonics. So on balance most general practitioners, two-thirds, were satisfied with the existing division between drugs freely available and drugs obtainable on prescription only. And among those who thought a change desirable most wanted an increase in restriction. This would probably add to their work and responsibility.

The influence of the doctor's age

Younger doctors were more likely to say they encouraged their patients to use appropriate self-treatment, although there was no difference in the conditions they regarded as appropriate for self-treatment. Eighty-two per cent of those under fifty said they did something to encourage self-treatment, 69% of older doctors. Also they had more often suggested that a patient should buy some item of medicine himself. Sixty-seven per cent of the younger doctors, those under 55, had suggested this at least once

[14] Balint, Michael; Hunt, John; Joyce, Dick; Marinker, Marshall and Woodcock, Jasper, 1970, *Treatment or Diagnosis*, p. 64.
[15] 'Are there any kinds of drugs that are only obtainable on prescription at the moment that you would like to see made freely available to the public?'
[16] 'Are there any kinds of drugs freely obtainable that you would like to see made available on prescription only?'

during the previous fortnight compared with 40% of the older doctors. The younger doctors were more in favour of people being encouraged to seek pharmacists' advice about health and medicines: over a third of them thought people could ask pharmacists for advice, less than a quarter of the older doctors. So younger doctors seem more in favour of self-treatment. They were also more likely to mention the general practitioner's role in the health education of patients. A fifth of the doctors under 40 thought that education of the patient by the general practitioner would reduce consultations for ailments people could self-treat.[17] The proportion fell to less than a twentieth of the doctors aged 60 or more.

Feeling they had a part to play in helping patients learn to cope with minor ailments effectively may have made younger doctors more tolerant of consultation for ailments that people could cope with alone. Thirty-nine per cent of the younger doctors thought that a quarter or more of their consultations were for these minor ailments, 56% of the older doctors. It may be that as doctors get older they become less tolerant of what they see as unnecessary consultations, and disenchanted with the small proportion of their patients who take up a large proportion of their time. But there may be a generation rather than just an age effect. More recent medical education may make doctors feel they have a wider role with greater emphasis on health education.

How was the age of the doctor related to his prescribing habits? Younger doctors, those under 50, wrote similar numbers of prescriptions per person on their list as older doctors wrote. Their prescribing costs, however, were more often higher than average. These results are shown in Table 43. Information obtained from the questionnaires of both adults and their doctors also suggests that younger doctors did not write more prescriptions per patient than older doctors. Patients of younger doctors had not taken more prescribed medicines than patients of older doctors. In addition there were no differences between the younger and older doctors in the proportion who thought they wrote a prescription at more than two-thirds of their consultations, but younger ones thought they wrote a higher proportion

[17] 'Do you think anything should be done to try and reduce the number of consultations which patients make for minor ailments which are self-limiting and can be self-treated? What?'

of prescriptions without seeing patients. (Sixteen per cent of those under 50 thought they wrote more than a fifth of their prescriptions in the absence of the patient, 6% of those aged 50 or more.)

Thus younger doctors are probably not more frequent but they are more expensive prescribers than older doctors. This may

TABLE 43   *Doctors' age and prescribing*

	Age of doctor	
Proportion of doctors whose averages were above the mean for:	*Under 50*	*50 or more*
Average number of prescriptions per person on N.H.S. list[a]	21%	17%
Average cost per prescription	54%	35%
Average cost per person on N.H.S. list	54%	42%
Number of doctors (= 100%)	200	119

[a] This distribution is very skewed, resulting in a small number of doctors having an average above the mean value.

be because they gained their initial training in therapeutics at a later date when drug manufacturers were producing more expensive and complex drugs. The younger doctors also relied on information from drug firms more than older doctors. Forty-eight per cent of doctors under 35 said that drug firms were their most important source of information about new drugs on the market. Twenty-four per cent of doctors aged between 35 and 59 said this, only 11% of those aged 60 or more. This information from drug firms generally advertises the newer, more complex, highly researched and therefore more expensive pharmaceutical products.

Variations with type of practice

The number of patients the doctor looked after[18] was related to his prescribing. Doctors with relatively few patients seemed to write more prescriptions per patient than those with larger lists.

[18] 'What is the approximate number of your N.H.S. patients? If you are in partnership please estimate the number you yourself look after.'

This is shown in Table 44. This variation in prescribing patterns with list size seems somewhat surprising in the light of the other finding that many doctors felt they would write fewer prescriptions if they had more time. In fact doctors with small lists were less likely to think this. Forty-two per cent of the doctors who

TABLE 44   *Doctors' prescribing and the number of patients looked after*

	Number of patients		
	Less than 2,000	2,000 < 3,000	3,000 or more
Proportion of doctors whose average number of prescriptions per patient was above average	29%	22%	13%
Number of doctors (= 100%)	49	158	108

looked after less than 2,000 patients thought they would write fewer prescriptions if they had more time, 50% of those with between 2,000 and 3,000 patients and 61% of those with 3,000 or more. These findings suggest that if doctors with larger lists had more time they might see their patients more often and would therefore not cut down their prescribing in the way they predict.

The assumption that the number of patients a doctor looks after reflects the pressure of his work is challenged by Mechanic. He concluded from his study: 'Apparently it is not the number of patients one cares for or how long one works that is most important, but rather the pressure patient load places on the mode of the doctor's practice.'[19] This helps to explain why in the present study the size of a doctor's list was not related to some other aspects of his work like the number of conditions doctors thought suitable for self-treatment, nor to doctors' encouragement or discouragement of self-medication.

The number of doctors in a practice did not appear to be related to their prescribing patterns nor to any of the questions about prescribing or self-treatment except that single-handed doctors had less often suggested during the previous two weeks that a

[19] Mechanic, David, 1970, 'Correlates of frustration among British general practitioners'.

patient should buy his own medicine. Thirty-five per cent of the single-handed had suggested this compared to 62% of those in partnership; a difference which persisted when age was held constant.

Some doctors working in partnership qualify for a group practice payment[20] in excess of the basic practice allowance. These doctors differed in several ways from other general practitioners. Not surprisingly they were more likely to feel that other doctors were the most helpful source of information about new drugs; 11% thought this compared with 3% of doctors not in group practice. They also had less contact with drug firm representatives, only 5% had seen ten or more in the previous four weeks, 14% of the others. Those doctors receiving group practice payments reported fewer trivial consultations than other doctors and fewer prescriptions written in the absence of the patient. Forty per cent thought they wrote fewer than a fifth of their prescriptions without seeing the patient; 55% of other doctors thought this. Fifty-six per cent of other doctors reported that a quarter or more of their consultations were for ailments people could treat themselves; fewer, 43%, of the doctors in group practice said this. There was no evidence of any differences in the extent or cost of their prescribing.

Summary and discussion

Most of the doctors in the study acknowledged that self-treatment was sometimes appropriate and necessary and half of them thought that a quarter or more of their consultations were for ailments people could treat or cope with themselves without seeing the doctor. The doctors who thought a high proportion of their consultations fell into this category were more likely than others to say they felt it was generally suitable for most adults to treat themselves for a number of specific conditions without seeing the doctor. This is shown in Table 45. These doctors were also less likely to discourage self-treatment. The patients of these doctors consulted their doctors rather less frequently than patients

[20] These are practices of three or more doctors working together in close association from a common main surgery which can provide an economic and efficient service by sharing ancillary staff, providing a twenty-four-hour cover and pooling their specialist knowledge.

of doctors who regarded only a small proportion of their consultations as inappropriate. This might suggest that their views on what was appropriate for self-treatment had been effectively communicated to patients. But the doctors' views on the appropri-

TABLE 45   *Some variations between general practitioners who said that their consultations were for ailments that could be self-treated*

	Proportion of consultations said to be for ailments people could self-treat			
	Less than 10%	10% < 25%	25% < 50%	50% or more
Proportion who regarded four or more of the six illness situations as suitable for self-treatment	7%	9%	9%	19%
Proportion who do something to discourage self-treatment	86%	73%	77%	61%
Proportion suggesting what should be done to try and reduce consultations for minor ailments:				
nothing	15%	12%	7%	9%
patient education by general practitioners	13%	20%	20%	4%
financial disincentives	13%	25%	35%	33%
Proportion who had seen ten or more drug firm representatives in 4 weeks	4%	6%	11%	14%
Number of doctors (= 100%)[a]	54	109	95	62

[a] Small numbers of doctors who gave inadequate answers to different questions have been excluded when calculating percentages.

ateness or otherwise of various conditions for self-treatment without consultation were unrelated to their patients' predictions about which of the same conditions they would consult the doctor and which they would treat themselves. Many other analyses relating the views and practices of doctors to the attitudes and habits of their particular patients also gave negative results. Both patients and doctors differed widely among themselves in their views on what was appropriate for consultation. In fact few doctors who thought half or more of their consultations inappropriate felt general practitioners should play a part in the health education of their patients in order to reduce the number of consultations for minor ailments which are self-limiting and can be self-treated. They were more likely to be in favour of some financial barrier between patients and doctors or between patients and prescribed medication. (See Table 45.) They had also seen more drug-firm representatives, but there was no difference between those doctors and others in the numbers or costs of the prescriptions they wrote.

The doctors' age did not appear to be related to the number of prescriptions they wrote but younger doctors tended to be more expensive prescribers. Size of list on the other hand was associated with relative frequency of prescribing and at first sight in an unexpected way; doctors looking after smaller numbers of patients wrote more prescriptions per patient. Many doctors obviously did not feel entirely happy about their prescribing patterns. More than half of them felt they would write fewer prescriptions if they had more time. This suggests that according to their own standards they felt they were giving prescriptions instead of more time-consuming forms of care. But the proportion who thought they would write fewer prescriptions if they had more time did not vary with their prescribing rates. It did however increase with the number of patients they looked after. Doctors' views of their own prescribing habits and possible feelings of anxiety about them may be related more to the absolute number of prescriptions they write rather than to their prescribing rate per person on their list.

Although a quarter of the doctors found drug firm literature or representatives their most helpful source of information about new drugs, and nearly half of them had seen five or more representatives in the last four weeks, neither of these possible indices of their exposure to, and reliance on, the pressure of the pharmaceutical industry appeared to be related to their prescribing levels or prescribing costs.

7

MEDICINES IN THE HOME

In 1968 people in England and Wales took home £152 million worth of medicines obtained on general practitioners' prescriptions. They also bought about £80 million worth of non-prescribed medicines from chemists' shops and other stores.[1] How many medicines are lying around in people's homes? The answer matters for economic and safety reasons. Prescribed medicines are expensive and the bulk of the cost is paid out of public expenditure. The average net ingredient cost of a prescription from a general practitioner in 1968 was £0·41, including the container and pharmacist's fee it was £0·57.

Many drugs can be dangerous. Apart from the 1,747 people who committed suicide with analgesic and soporific drugs in 1967 there were 750 accidental deaths caused by these drugs and another 67 caused by other drugs.[2] Three per cent of such accidental deaths occurred to children under fifteen. In addition there were a number of unsuccessful suicide attempts by drug overdose. Other people became ill but did not die as a result of accidents. The deaths caused by drugs probably represent only a small proportion of the suffering caused by the storage of medicines in people's homes.

Sedative drugs seem readily obtainable from general practitioners, analgesics are available without prescription and in any quantity, from chemists' shops. People could not identify sufficiently for us to classify a quarter of the prescribed medicines they were taking currently, so the chances of muddling them up with old medicines and of taking the wrong sort must be fairly high. Many tablets are attractive to young children and, if they are

[1] Department of Health and Social Security, 1969, *Annual Report for 1968*, p. 99; Office of Health Economics, 1968, *Without Prescription*, p. 4.
[2] Registrar General, 1968, *Statistical Review of England and Wales for the year 1967*, pp. 38 and 167.

not kept locked up, children may find and eat them. Another newer potential hazard is that of the teenager experimenting with drugs and finding the family medicine collection a useful source of supply.

Some health authorities have tried to reduce the quantity of drugs in people's homes by displaying posters warning of the dangers and inviting people to return their unused medicines to chemists' shops or destroy them. Such a scheme was introduced in Hartlepool during March 1967.[3] During one week 43,554 tablets and capsules were handed in of which 36,242 were identified. A fifth of these were sedatives, tranquillisers or hypnotics, an eighth analgesics. It was estimated that these were from only 500 homes—an average of nearly 90 tablets in each. These 500 households however were not representative of all households. The present survey tried to look at the medicines kept in a national sample of households.[4]

Methods

Information was collected about the medicines in 686 households in the fourteen study areas. The information was normally collected from the housewife after the interview with the adult and about any children. This procedure was found to be advantageous because by this time the interviewer had gained the confidence of the informant and his family who then did not mind talking about their medicine collection. Each individual container of medicine was listed and then a series of questions was asked about each one. Interviewers were instructed to ask about medicines kept in every room of the house as well as in handbags and cars. If possible the interviewer went from room to room with the informant because seeing the medicines made recording easier and more accurate. Even so it is possible that people had medicines that were not recorded at the interview. If a household had a large number of medicines the interview took a long time and informants may have foreseen this and discussed only some of their medicines.

3 Nicholson, W. A., 1967, 'Collection of unwanted drugs from private homes'.
4 Details of the sample are given in Appendix I.

Unidentified medicines

A great effort was made in this part of the survey to identify all the tablets found. This was possible here, though not on the survey of what people were currently taking, because so many of the medicines were not in use.

Nine per cent of the medicines in people's homes were tablets which the informant could not identify adequately for us to classify. A sample was obtained for 80% of these. For 11% the interviewer did not ask for one, 4% of the tablets were being taken and for the remaining 5% a sample was refused. So nearly four hundred tablets were sent to the Poisons Unit at Guy's Hospital in London for identification because people could not identify them. Eighty per cent of those sent were identified. Of these 20% were central nervous system drugs, 16% analgesics, 16% cardio-vascular and genito-urinary preparations, 10% antibiotics, 8% iron and vitamins. Drugs acting on the central nervous system and analgesics are those which are most often responsible for accidents and suicide. They also make up a large part of those medicines which are in people's homes and are unidentifiable except by the expert.

In addition, to see whether tablets were in fact correctly identified by informants a random sample of 150 tablets was collected. Fifteen others were refused, ten could not be collected as they formed part of a current course of medication. The Poisons Unit were unable to identify 22% of those collected. Of the 117 they identified, 113 (97%) had been correctly described by the informant. No attempt was made to collect samples of liquids and creams for identification.

The medicines in people's homes

All of the 686 households except six, 1%, had some medicines in them. A tenth had twenty or more. On average the households had 10·3 different items. Nearly all homes, 94%, had some non-prescribed medicines; fewer, 73%, had prescribed ones. Table 46 shows the proportions of households with different numbers of prescribed and non-prescribed medicines.

Apart from classifying the medicines according to whether they had been prescribed by a doctor or not, each one was

TABLE 46   *Numbers of medicines (prescribed and non-prescribed) in households*

	Type of medicine		
	Prescribed	Non-prescribed	All medicines
Number of medicines:	%	%	%
None	27	6	1
1–9	68	69	59
10 or more	5	25	40
Mean number of medicines	3·0	7·3	10·3
Number of households (= 100%)	684	686	686

assigned to a group with the pharmacological classification devised for the study by Jasper Woodcock.[5] As previous chapters have shown, analgesics were the most commonly taken kind of medicine; they were also the kind most often found in people's homes. Table 47 shows the proportions of households with the different kinds of medicines. Most, 85%, had analgesics; a fifth had some kind of sedative, sleeping tablet or tranquilliser. Two-fifths of the households had at least one container of medicine that the informant could not identify. This proportion was reduced to three-tenths by the identification of the collected samples of tablets.[6] Twenty-eight per cent of the medicines in people's homes had been prescribed by a doctor. Table 48 shows how the prescribed and non-prescribed medicines differed. Among the prescribed, the largest group was those drugs acting on the central nervous system, three-fifths of which were sedatives, tranquillisers and sleeping tablets. They made up 14% of the prescribed items.

Where they were kept

Of the 686 homes only two had any medicines locked up with the key elsewhere than in the lock. The most popular place for

[5] This was described in Chapter 3.
[6] Most of these households had only one unidentified drug. The 351 medicines that remained unidentified amounted to only 5% of the total of 7,059 items of medicine found in the 686 homes.

Medicines in the Home

TABLE 47   *Proportions of households with different kinds of medicines in them*

	Proportion with medicine
	%
Preparations acting on the digestive system	
Laxatives	43
Indigestion remedies	35
Tonics	6
Anti-diarrhoeals	8
Preparations acting on the respiratory system and ears, nose and throat	
Cough and lower respiratory preparations	35
Upper respiratory and nose preparations	33
Antihistamines and cold remedies	7
Mouth and throat preparations	23
Ear preparations	6
Preparations acting on the nervous system	
Analgesics and antipyretics	85
Sedatives, sleeping tablets, tranquillisers	20
Antidepressives, stimulants	7
Antinauseants, travel sickness tablets	6
Preparations acting systemically on infections	
Antibiotics	13
Preparations affecting metabolism, nutrition and blood	
Iron and vitamins	29
Preparations used in rheumatic diseases	
Embrocations, rubs, counter irritants	27
Anti-rheumatics, corticosteroids	7
Preparations acting on eye	
Eye drops and creams	22
Preparations acting on the skin	
Simple skin creams	48
Other skin creams	54
Dressings	33
Something unidentified	29
No medicines	1
Total number of households (= 100%)	686

TABLE 48   *Therapeutic group distribution of the medicines found in people's homes*

Therapeutic group (D.H.S.S.)	Non-prescribed medicines	Prescribed medicines	All medicines in the homes
	%	%	%
Preparations acting on the digestive system (06, 08, 19, 60, 69)	15·8	8·4	13·9
Preparations acting on the cardio-vascular and genito-urinary systems and diuretics (6X, 5y)	0·2	6·4	1·8
Preparations acting on the lower respiratory system (05)	4·3	8·7	5·4
Preparations acting on the nervous system:			
Analgesics and antipyretics (01)	18·5	10·3	16·2
Acting on CNS (30, 39, 3X, 3y)	1·3	13·9	4·5
Preparations acting systemically on infections and immunological preparations (6y)	0·1	5·8	1·6
Preparations affecting metabolism, nutrition and blood (10, 1X, 1y, 50, 5X)	4·1	11·0	5·9
Preparations used in rheumatic diseases (03, 59)	4·7	6·1	5·1
Preparations affecting allergic reactions (2y)	0·4	2·2	0·9
Preparations acting on ear, nose and throat (04, 20, 2X)	10·5	8·2	9·8
Preparations acting on the eye (29)	2·8	4·0	3·1
Preparations acting on the skin (02, 49, 40, 4X, 4y)	27·4	12·8	23·7
Medicinal food, drink etc. (79, 70, 7X)	2·0	0·4	1·6
Surgical clothing and dressings (07, 89)	7·7	1·5	6·2
Others not elsewhere classifiable (8X)	0·2	0·3	0·3
Total number of medicines (= 100%)	4,922	1,714	6,708 [a]

[a] The sum totals of the first two columns do not equal that of the last column because for some medicines inadequate information was obtained about whether or not they were prescribed.

keeping medicines was the kitchen. Forty-four per cent of the medicines were kept there, 23% in the bathroom, 16% in a living room and 11% in an adult's bedroom. Less than 0·5% of all the medicines were kept in a bedroom where children slept. Six per cent of medicines were kept in other places such as cars and handbags.

Social class differences

Chapter 5 showed that the small differences in the extent of medicine taking between social classes were apparently explained by levels of symptom reporting. Therefore we did not expect to find much difference in the numbers of medicines people kept in their homes. However Table 49 shows a trend: the higher social

TABLE 49 *Social class and numbers of medicines in the home*

	Social class						
	I	II	III Skilled	III	IV	V	*All*
	Profes-sional	Inter-mediate	non-manual	Skilled manual	Semi-skilled	Un-skilled	*house-holds*
Proportion of households with:							
Ten or more non-prescribed medicines	31%	34%	22%	24%	22%	20%	25%
Four or more prescribed medicines	31%	38%	31%	33%	27%	46%	33%
Ten or more medicines altogether	50%	47%	40%	39%	36%	32%	40%
Mean number of medicines	11·0	11·8	9·6	10·2	9·3	8·3	10·3
Number of households (= 100%)	26	122	89	233	114	41	625

classes having more medicines in their homes than the lower classes. Half the Social Class I households[7] had ten or more items of medicine, less than a third of the Social Class V homes. The professional and intermediate group had an average of 11·7 items,

[7] Households were classified by the occupation of the sample adult, as described in Appendix VIII.

the semi-skilled and unskilled 9·1. When the medicines were grouped into prescribed and non-prescribed it was found that this trend existed for non-prescribed medicines only, not for prescribed ones.

These data on social class differences suggest variations in the buying, although not the taking, patterns of people in different social classes. Prescribed medicines are cheaply or freely available and were found in similar quantities in all households. Non-prescribed medicines are generally more expensive to obtain and were found in smaller quantities in the homes of the less well-off social classes. As the households in the higher social classes had more non-prescribed medicines they might be expected to be more likely to have the kinds of medicines which are largely non-prescribed like analgesics, digestive system remedies, simple skin creams and respiratory preparations. However, they did not. This suggests that people in the lower social classes are more likely to have only one brand of these commonly found over-the-counter medicines whereas middle-class people tend to have more than one. Poorer people are more likely to buy them in smaller quantities and use up any remainder before buying a new supply or switching to a different brand.

The differences between social classes in the kinds of prescribed medicines they had in their homes were largely restricted to a few medicines which were found in a minority of households. Social Class I and II households were more likely to have anti-diar-rhoeals, and antihistamines and cold remedies. They were also more likely to have the therapeutic skin creams which are mostly obtained on prescription. For example, 38% of the Social Class I and II homes had some kind of antibiotic, antiseptic, fungicidal or keratolytic ointment or powder compared to 24% of the other households. Non-manual workers' homes had on average fewer medicines that the informant could not identify than manual workers' homes; 0·7 each compared with 1·0.

Social Class I households were nearly twice as likely as any other group to keep most of their medicines in the bathroom. Over half of them did so but the proportion fell to under a tenth of the Social Class V households, who would be less likely to have a bathroom at all. Opposite trends were found for both the kitchen and living room. The lower down the social class scale structure the more likely people were to keep most of their medicines in the kitchen or living room. Details are given in Table 50. These differences probably reflect housing conditions such as possession and size of bathrooms, the extent of fitted furniture in homes and the ways in which the main cooking and living areas are used. No information was collected about this.

TABLE 50   *Social class and main room in which medicines kept*

	Social class						
	I	II	III Skilled non-manual	III Skilled manual	IV Semi-skilled	V Un-skilled	*All homes*
	Profes-sional	Inter-mediate					
Room where majority of medicines kept:	%	%	%	%	%	%	%
Bathroom	54	29	23	18	12	7	20
Kitchen	20	32	42	48	47	38	42
Living room	—	8	10	17	21	34	16
Bedroom	14	14	12	9	4	6	9
Other and no special place	12	17	13	8	16	15	13
Number of house-holds (= 100%)	25	121	86	225	107	41	666[a]

[a] This figure is more than the sum of the different social classes because the households of people who gave inadequate information about their occupation, or who were students or in the armed forces are excluded from the social class breakdown.

Area differences

We found few differences between either urban and rural areas or those north and south of the Bristol/Wash line, in the numbers or the kinds of medicines that were taken or used during a two-week period. Neither were there differences in the proportions of people who had had a consultation or prescription or who reported different numbers and kinds of symptoms.[8] The numbers of medicines kept in homes in urban and rural areas did not differ. However there were differences between homes in the north and south. Households in the south had on average more items of both

[8] Area differences were somewhat confounded by variations in the time of the year at which people were interviewed. This is discussed in Appendix IV.

prescribed and non-prescribed medicines than those in the north. Households in the northern areas had an average of 9·4 items, those in the south an average of 11·2. A similar difference existed between the areas for the different social classes (see Table 51).

TABLE 51   *Social class differences north and south of the Bristol/Wash line in the numbers of medicines in the home*

	Average number of medicines in households		
	Social class		
	I and II Professional and intermediate	III Skilled	IV and V Semi-skilled and unskilled
North	11·3 (76)	8·9 (183)	8·3 (90)
South	12·1 (72)	11·5 (139)	10·1 (65)

The figures in brackets are the numbers of households for which means were calculated.

Differences related to size and composition of household

As could be expected the more people there were in a household the more medicines there were in general. The trend, which seemed to level off, or even fall, at six-person households is shown in Table 52. However the number of items per head fell with increasing household size from eight each for people living alone to less than two each for those living in six person or larger

TABLE 52   *Relationship between size of household and the number of medicines kept*

	Number of people in household					
	1	2	3	4	5	6 or more
Proportion of households with ten or more medicines	26%	34%	44%	50%	53%	38%
Mean number of medicines	7·5	9·2	10·7	11·9	12·6	10·8
Number of households (= 100%)	106	194	126	135	66	42

households. Obviously people in the same household often share each other's medicines. When asked who the medicines had been obtained for, a third of all the medicines in peoples' homes and nearly half the non-prescribed ones were said to be for general use. One in seven of those obtained for a particular person had also been used by someone else and this proportion was 20% of non-prescribed medicines and 6% of prescribed ones.

Households with one or more children under fifteen had on average more of both prescribed and non-prescribed medicines than childless homes. They had an average of 3·7 prescribed items compared with the 2·6 of childless homes, and 9·0 non-prescribed items compared with 6·3.⁹ Only a quarter of the households with children living in them did not have any prescribed medicines. As the homes with children in had so many more items of medicine they were more likely to have different kinds of medicines. The only kinds of medicines that they were less likely to have than those without children were preparations acting on the central nervous system like sleeping tablets and genito-urinary and cardio-vascular medicines. These drugs are taken mostly by people aged 45 or over who are less likely than younger adults to live in households with young children. Households with children in them were more likely to keep most of their medicines in the kitchen than childless homes. They were less likely to keep most of them in living rooms and bedrooms. Fifty-four per cent of homes with children kept most in the kitchen, 40% of the others.

Hoarding

How long had the medicines been in people's homes and how recently had they used them? Just over a fifth of all the items had been obtained during the month before the interview, another third during the five months prior to that. Twenty-nine per cent of all the medicines had been in people's homes for a year or more. Non-prescribed medicines had been hoarded for longer: 32% had been obtained a year or more ago compared with 22% of prescribed medicines. Table 53 shows the proportions of different kinds of medicines which had been kept for a year or

⁹ When similar sized households are compared those with children still had more medicines than those with no children.

TABLE 53 *Hoarding different types of medicine*

	Type of medicine										
	Analgesics	Lower respiratory	Nutrition and metabolism	Central nervous system	Digestive system	Ear, nose and throat preparation	Skin	Rheumatic diseases	Unidentified medicines	Others	All medicines
Proportion that had been obtained a year or more before the interview	12%	15%	17%	23%	30%	36%	41%	43%	25%	33%	29%
Last used:	%	%	%	%	%	%	%	%	%	%	%
Less than 1 month ago	62	47	61	59	47	30	40	40	56	43	47
1 month but less than 6 months ago	22	31	18	14	20	29	20	19	16	21	21
6 months but less than a year ago	6	10	7	8	9	14	13	12	8	9	10
1 year or more ago	6	10	12	16	19	24	24	27	18	20	18
Not been used at all	4	2	2	3	5	3	3	2	2	7	4
Total number of medicines (= 100%)[a]	1,088	363	397	302	931	660	1,590	344	351	1,033	7,059

[a] Small numbers for which inadequate information was obtained have been omitted when calculating percentages.

more. Aspirin and other pain-killers were the kind that were least likely to have been in people's homes for a long time, but they are of course the most commonly taken drugs, so supplies would be used up more quickly. Skin preparations and medicines for rheumatic diseases (85% of which were local applications) were the kinds of medicine most likely to have been obtained more than a year before. These were also the medicines that were least likely to have been used during the previous year; 73% had been used in this period compared with 81% of all other medicines. The length of time since different kinds of medicines had been taken is also shown at Table 53. As can be seen this is related to how long ago the medicines had been obtained. Ninety per cent of analgesics had been used during the previous year compared with 81% of the central nervous system drugs and 71% of the rheumatic preparations. Prescribed medicines had been used more recently than non-prescribed. Fifty-five per cent of the prescribed items had been used during the previous month, but less, 44%, of the non-prescribed.

Waste [10]

People reported that 45% of the prescribed medicines in their homes had not been used at all during the month before the interview, 25% during the previous six months. If we assume that most drugs are either prescribed for a specific episode of sickness or for a chronic long-term disorder then it would appear that all these prescribed medicines that had not been used for a month are either never used up, or are used for subsequent episodes when the medicine may have deteriorated. There are of course some conditions like asthma, hay fever, some skin troubles and sleeplessness which may occur sporadically and for which people may keep drugs in case they need them. Table 54 shows the proportion of different kinds of prescribed medicines that people had not used during the month and during the six months before the interview. Nearly half the antibiotics had not been used during the previous month. It is important that these drugs are taken as a complete course of medication but, because they are quickly effective in relieving symptoms of infections, people are tempted to stop taking them before they have finished the

10 This section on waste refers only to prescribed medicines.

TABLE 54　*Proportions of different types of prescribed medicines that had not been used during the month before the interview*

	Types of prescribed medicines												
		Upper respiratory	Skin preparations	Antibiotics	Lower respiratory	Digestive system	Rheumatic diseases	Analgesics	Central nervous system	Nutrition and metabolism	Cardio-vascular and genito-urinary	Others	All types
Proportion that had not been used during the month before interview		78%	58%	48%	44%	42%	41%	40%	32%	28%	23%	49%	45%
Proportion that had not been used during the 6 months before interview		46%	33%	23%	19%	20%	25%	17%	20%	15%	13%	31%	25%
Number of items (= 100%)		138	215	94	144	142	105	172	232	183	107	407	1,939

complete course. This can lead to relapse. Our data suggest that
in fact patients are not finishing courses of antibiotics that are
prescribed for them, and part of many of the medicines prescribed
by doctors and largely paid for by the National Health Service
are left unused in people's homes.

What proportion of the originally prescribed quantity is left
in these containers? At the interview the proportion left in the
container was estimated with the help of the respondent. This
measure is obviously not exact but gives a general idea of how
full the containers were. Table 55 shows that there were similar

TABLE 55   *Estimated proportion of prescribed medicines left in containers at the*
time of interview

	Proportion of prescribed medicines
	%
Proportion left:	
Less than $\frac{1}{4}$	21
$\frac{1}{4}$ but less than $\frac{1}{2}$	28
$\frac{1}{2}$ but less than $\frac{3}{4}$	25
$\frac{3}{4}$ or more	26
Number of items (= 100%)	1,931

proportions of medicines falling into each of the four categories.
On average the containers were estimated to be half full. There
were no differences between different kinds of medicines. A look
at the proportion of medicine left in containers that had not been
used for different lengths of time suggests that prescribed medicines are hoarded without people really intending to use them
again in the near future. Thirty-five per cent of containers with
medicines that had not been used for a year or more were three-
quarters or more full, compared with 22% of more recently
used ones. That medicines that had been used more recently were
in emptier containers is probably a reflection of the frequency
with which they were used. People may also be more reluctant
to throw away a container that has a substantial quantity of
medicine left in it.

Four hundred and forty-eight prescribed medicines had been obtained more than a month but less than a year before the interview and had not been used during the previous month. If this is taken as the number wasted but still kept during an eleven-month period, the estimated number for twelve months is 489. This is an average of 0·71 for each household in the survey. In 1966[11] there were an estimated 17·0 million households in England, Wales and Scotland. Thus the estimated number of these medicines in households in Great Britain is 12·1 million. In 1968 the average net ingredient cost per prescription was £0·43. It was estimated that the medicine containers were on average half full. This suggests that the ingredient cost of all these prescribed medicines amounts to £2·7 million. (This assumes that the medicines which were not used had the same average costs as all prescriptions.) As a proportion of the total ingredient cost of medicines dispensed in 1968[12] this represents 2·1%. If only those medicines not taken for six months or longer are counted as wasted this proportion falls to 0·9%. These estimates do not include of course any measure of those prescribed medicines which were thrown away.

Some idea of how many are thrown away can be gained from the answers to questions about what the adults had done with the prescriptions they had obtained during the two weeks before interview. If they were still using the medicine at the time of the interview they were asked 'What will you do with any that is left?'; if they had already stopped taking it, 'What have you done with what is left?' People thought they would use up four-fifths of the medicines they were still taking, they would throw away 12% and keep only 8%. Of those medicines which people had stopped taking, fewer, two-fifths, were finished up 39% were kept and might be used later, 16% had been thrown away. If we assume from this that people threw away some of about 13% of the medicine they obtained on prescription and that the containers were a third full when they did so, this means that another 4·3% of all prescribed medicines are wasted, making a total of between 5·2% and 6·4% (depending on the assumptions

[11] General Register Office, 1967, *Sample Census 1966*, p. 2.
[12] Department of Health and Social Security, 1969, *Annual Report for 1968*; and Scottish Home and Health Department, 1969, *Health and Welfare Services in Scotland, Report for 1968*.

made about the waste of medicines still in the home). This is equivalent to between £6·7 and £8·2 million (around 250 to 300 times the cost of this study).

Availability and advice

The survey has shown that there were more than twice as many non-prescribed as prescribed medicines readily available for use in people's homes: an average of 7·3 non-prescribed and 3·0 prescribed ones. New supplies of non-prescribed medicines are also easier to obtain as they can be purchased from chemist shops as well as other stores without a prescription. More than half, 57%, of the adults regarded the chemist as a good person to ask for advice when not feeling well.[13] As well as thinking that the chemist was an appropriate source of advice about medicines more people found it quicker and easier to get to a chemist's shop than to get to a doctor's surgery:[14] 48% compared with 21%. The rest found their doctor and a chemist's shop equally accessible. Chemists' shops are of course open all day long whereas most doctors' surgery sessions are restricted to a morning and afternoon/evening period.

To get a prescription people first have to contact the doctor or the surgery or ask the doctor to call. Three-quarters of the adults lived less than fifteen minutes journey from the surgery but added to that was the wait, which for half of them was fifteen minutes or more. A survey of a similar population in 1964[15] found that more, 80%, of adults lived less than fifteen minutes journey from their doctor's surgery. This suggests that the growth in group practices and health centres may have increased the average journey time to doctors' surgeries.

Maddock[16] has reported on the declining number of chemists' shops which he also attributes to the trend for doctors to work together in larger groups. Included in the time taken to obtain a prescription is the dispensing time: the patient usually has to

---

[13] 'In general do you think a chemist is a good person to ask for advice when you are not feeling well?'
[14] 'Which is the quickest and easiest to get to: your doctor's surgery or a chemist shop?'
[15] Cartwright, Ann, 1967, *Patients and their Doctors*, p. 106.
[16] Maddock, D. H., 1971, Masters thesis to Welsh School of Pharmacy; reported in *Guardian*, 19 April.

visit a chemist's shop to get the medicine and wait for it to be made up. The travelling time may not be affected by a decrease in chemists' shops as it is likely to be those with no nearby surgery that have to close through lack of business. The decrease may however affect the availability of over-the-counter medicines although these are increasingly available from other retail stores.

How often do people buy over-the-counter medicines and how do they go about it? To find out about this additional questions were asked about all those non-prescribed medicines in people's homes that had been bought during the month before the interview. There were 787 of them, an average of 1·1 per household. This sample does not of course include those that had been bought and completely used up. The majority, 79%, had been bought from a chemist's shop, 17% from general or other stores, only 4% from supermarkets. Three-quarters of all the medicines had been bought by the informants personally, and they were asked whether or not they had had that medicine before and if not whether they wanted advice about what to buy. Nine-tenths of the medicines had been bought before so only a small number of medicines were bought for which the person wanted advice. That only a minority of people going into chemists' shops seek advice about the non-prescribed medicines they buy, is also suggested by a question asked of the sample of adults[17] about each of the non-prescribed items they had taken. For only 6% of the medicines was the chemist reported to have been the first person who suggested that particular medicine. Table 56 shows however that a fifth of the non-prescribed medicines taken by adults had been suggested by a doctor or other para-medical personnel such as dentists, district nurses and pharmacists. Parents and grandparents were the people most often mentioned from whom advice about self-medication was obtained, and friends, neighbours and people at work apparently had more influence than husbands and wives. Of those medicines taken by married people less than a tenth were reported to have first been suggested by a spouse. Impersonal sources of ideas, such as advertising and reading about which medicines to use, were named for about a tenth of the medicines.

[17] 'Who or what first gave you the idea?'

TABLE 56   *Who or what first gave adults the idea of using the non-prescribed medicines they had taken*

Who or what first gave idea:	%
Spouse	7
Parents/grandparents	18
Other relatives	5
Friends, etc.	13
Doctor	10
Para-medical people	4
Chemist	6
Advertising	8
Can't remember, etc.	22
Other, including reading	7
Number of medicines (= 100%)	1,902

Summary

This chapter has discussed the results from a survey of the medicines kept in a sample of households in England, Wales and Scotland. Ninety-nine per cent of these homes had one or more medicines. The average number of items was 10·3; 3·0 prescribed and 7·3 non-prescribed. Nearly all had some kind of analgesic and skin cream. A fifth of the households had sedatives, tranquillisers or sleeping tablets and two-fifths had one item or more that the informant could not identify. Only two of the 686 homes surveyed had any medicines locked up at the time of inquiry. Medicines were most commonly kept in the kitchen.

Although there were no geographical or social-class differences in the extent of the *use* of medicines there were variations in the numbers people kept in their homes. Households in the study areas south of the Bristol/Wash line had on average more of both prescribed and non-prescribed medicines than those to the north. Middle-class homes had more non-prescribed, though not prescribed items, than working-class homes.

In general the larger the household, the more medicines there were kept in it. Homes with children under fifteen living in them had both more prescribed and non-prescribed medicines than childless homes, but they were less likely to have drugs acting on the central nervous system, or genito-urinary and cardio-vascular preparations.

Three-tenths of the medicines had been obtained a year or more before the interview. A fifth of all of them had not been taken during the previous year. Analgesics, the most commonly taken type of medicine, were the least likely to have been obtained as long ago as that, but nearly a quarter of drugs acting on the central nervous system had been in the home for a year or more.

Forty-four per cent of the non-prescribed medicines had been used by someone in the household during the previous month. More, 55%, of prescribed items had been taken in this time. Prescribed medicines obtained in the last year but not taken recently account for between 0·9% and 2·1% of the cost of prescribed ingredients. Medicines thrown away were estimated at 4·3% making a total of between 5·2% and 6·4% which could be regarded as wasted, or at least not taken according to the doctor's instructions.

8

PATTERNS IN THE USE OF COMMONLY TAKEN MEDICINES

Previous chapters have described the extent of use of different kinds of medicines and variations in the ways in which they were used. The relationships of age, sex, social class and various attitudes with the numbers of both prescribed and non-prescribed medicines taken have been discussed. This chapter looks at the data from a different perspective. It describes and discusses the different patterns of use of the most commonly taken medicines, starting with analgesics.

Analgesics[1]

Over 570 adults, 41% of the sample, said in response to the check list of medicines that they had taken 'aspirin or other pain-killers' during the two weeks before the interview. Eight per cent of these people had taken more than one brand or type of pain-killer. Not surprisingly the most common complaint for which these analgesics were taken was headache. Fifty-eight per cent were taken for that or for migraine, 14% for musculoskeletal symptoms or conditions like rheumatism, arthritis and backache, 12% for respiratory conditions and symptoms such as colds and sore throats. Analgesics had been given to 18% of the children during the two-week period. A third of these had been given to children for headache or migraine, a quarter for respiratory symptoms.

Women more often reported the symptoms for which analgesics were taken than men. They had more headaches; 46% reported

[1] Throughout this chapter when the people taking aspirins, for example, are identified, these are the people who in the interview said at the check list that they had taken 'aspirin or other pain-killers'. On the other hand when the aspirins are discussed they are the medicines that were coded as such in the pharmacological classification. The two classifications are compared in Appendix III.

them compared with 30% of the men, backaches, 23% and 18%, and joint and muscle pains, 32% and 26%. In addition they had period pains. Not surprisingly women were more likely than men to have taken pain-killers. Half the women and a third of the men had taken some kind of analgesic during the two-week period. There was no difference between the proportions of boys and girls who had taken them, although there were age differences. Children aged between 5 and 9 were less likely to have been given analgesics than children of other ages. The proportions were 19% of children under 5, 12% of those aged 5–9 and 24% of those aged 10 to 14.

Pain-killers were different from most other types of medicines, except skin creams, in that they were reported as having been taken by more younger than older adults in the two-week period. Forty-six per cent of the people between 21 and 54 reported taking pain-killers, 32% of people who were 55 or older. And the younger adults in the study more frequently reported some of the symptoms for which pain-killers are taken than did older people.

In Chapter 2 we showed that the reported prevalence of headaches, sore throats, 'women's complaints' and colds tended to decline with increasing age. Older people more often reported aches and pains in the joints, muscles and limbs than younger people but backache did not vary with age.[2] It seems that the extent of aspirin taking among younger adults is related to a higher incidence of minor symptoms and conditions. But people's perceptions of symptoms vary and taking a specific course of action such as medication for a symptom may increase a person's remembrance of it. A minor headache for which aspirin was taken may be more easily recalled than one for which nothing was done. It is possible therefore that younger people are more likely to take medicine for their minor symptoms than older people, and the process of medication leads to greater recall and reporting of these symptoms. It is not possible to test this hypothesis—that there is a difference in recall of treated and untreated symptoms that contributes to the age variations in reported symptoms—because of course we have information about only the reported ones.

Chapter 2 showed that the symptoms reported by younger

[2] Similar age patterns were found on another study. Wadsworth, M. E. J., Butterfield, W. J. H. and Blaney, R., 1971. *Health and Sickness: the Choice of Treatment*, p. 62.

people were no more likely to have been medicated than those of older people. This is also suggested by their answers to a question asking whether they agreed with the statement 'it is only sensible to take aspirins or something like that whenever you get a headache'. Three-fifths of the adults agreed but there were no differences between the age groups. Not unexpectedly agreement with this statement was related to aspirin taking. Half the people who agreed had taken an analgesic during the two-week period compared with just over a quarter of those who felt neutral or disagreed. They did not differ however in their consumption of prescribed medicines.

As Chapter 5 showed there were no social-class differences in the extent of either prescribed or non-prescribed medication. Neither were there variations in the proportions of people who had taken analgesics. This is similar to the findings of Elder and Acheson.[3] Their study in New Haven of social class and behaviour in response to symptoms of osteoarthrosis, a common complaint, concluded that 'heat and aspirin, the most common remedies used, seemed to be part of the common culture, as they were used by all social classes both with and without physicians' endorsements'. In fact the decision to take analgesics is one which is nearly always made without the help of a doctor. Four per cent of those taken by the children and 16% of those taken by adults were prescribed, although another 10% of non-prescribed ones had first been suggested by a doctor. Two-fifths of the prescribed analgesics were taken for rheumatism and arthritis compared with less than a tenth of the non-prescribed ones.

One reason why some people may take prescribed rather than non-prescribed analgesics is that they are sometimes cheaper. People aged 65 or over were more likely to get their analgesics on prescription. Eighteen per cent of those taken by older people were prescribed, only 8% of those taken by younger people. This difference may be explained in part by the fact that older people are not charged for prescriptions.

Prescribed and non-prescribed analgesics differed greatly in the frequency with which they had been used. Only a tenth of the non-prescribed ones had been taken ten or more times during the two-week period compared with seven-tenths of the pre-

[3] Elder, Ruth and Acheson, Roy M., 1970, 'Social class and behaviour in response to symptoms of osteoarthrosis'.

scribed ones. Many of those taken frequently also seemed to be taken over long periods. Sixty-three per cent of the prescribed pain-killers that had been taken ten or more times in the fortnight had first been prescribed a year or more before the interview, 40% of those taken less frequently.

The general picture that emerges from this is that younger adults take aspirin for their minor self-limiting symptoms and conditions. They are self-prescribed and taken comparatively irregularly and infrequently. However as people get older they take analgesics for the relief of chronic conditions like rheumatism and arthritis. They are more likely to get these medicines from the doctor and to take them frequently. These various trends lead to a different age pattern in the taking of analgesics in a twenty-four-hour period. Over this time rather more older than younger people had taken them: 17% of those aged 65 or more, 13% of those under 65.

Creams, ointments and liquids for the skin

Fourteen per cent of the adults had used at least one kind of skin preparation during the two-week period. More than half, 54%, had been taken for diseases and symptoms of the skin, 14% for prevention or protection, 19% for cuts, burns and stings and 6% for circulatory conditions like chilblains and varicose ulcers. Three-tenths of the adults' skin medicaments were prescribed. Most of these, four-fifths, were for skin diseases and symptoms. Few, less than a tenth, of the skin preparations they used for accidents or for prevention or protection had been prescribed.

Like analgesics, skin medicaments were used more by the younger age groups than the older. Table 57 shows the general downward trend in the reporting of skin ailments with increasing age. As can be seen the use of skin preparations followed a similar pattern. Twenty per cent of the 21–24 age group reported using them, 11% of the people 75 and over. More women than men had used skin medicines, 16% compared with 12%, although there were no differences between the proportions of men and women reporting rashes, itches, cuts, bruises or other skin trouble. So women are more likely to treat their skin conditions than men, possibly for cosmetic reasons.

Skin preparations were the kind of medicine most commonly

TABLE 57 *Age and the reporting of skin conditions and the use of skin medicaments*

	Children				Adults						
	Less than 2	2–4	5–9	10–14	21–24	25–34	35–44	45–54	55–64	65–74	75+
Proportion reporting rashes, itches or other skin trouble	19%	10%	12%	11%	22%	17%	13%	17%	7%	10%	6%
Proportion reporting burns, bruises, cuts, etc.	7%	27%	20%	7%	14%	11%	9%	12%	9%	2%	3%
Proportion who had used skin medicaments	38%	26%	18%	9%	20%	17%	12%	17%	11%	13%	11%
Number of people (= 100%)	68	113	169	169	81	230	289	269	258	194	87

used by the children. There was a trend from 38% of the babies under 2 having them applied down to 9% of those aged 10 to 14. There was a similar variation in the reporting of rashes, itches and other skin troubles, although the 2 to 9 age group were reported as having three times as many cuts and bruises as the babies and older children, 23% compared with 7%. Thirty-nine per cent of the skin preparations used by children had been applied for skin diseases, including nappy rash, 36% for cuts and other accidents and 17% for preventive purposes. A fifth of the children's skin medicaments were prescribed.

Medicines acting on the digestive system

A quarter of the sample of adults had taken some kind of remedy acting on the digestive system during the two-week period. The most commonly taken were indigestion remedies; 14% had used these, compared to 9% using laxatives and 8% health salts. In fact nearly all the health salts had a mainly laxative action and were classified as such in the pharmacological classification. Sixty-one per cent of the laxatives described by people as 'laxatives' had been taken specifically to relieve constipation, compared with 27% of those thought of as 'health salts'. Nearly all the rest of the 'laxatives', 33%, were taken to prevent constipation, and 18% of the 'health salts' for the same reason. Less than a tenth of the medicines with a laxative action taken by the adults were precribed by a doctor, so most of these medicines were taken on a person's own initiative. A quarter of the non-prescribed ones were said to have been first suggested by parents or grandparents, compared with less than a fifth of other sorts of non-prescribed medicines. More than half (55%) of the medicines described as 'health salts' were taken for reasons other than as a laxative, for example to relieve rheumatism or to promote general health. It is likely that many people do not realise the laxative action of health salts.

Bowel habits seem to be something not well understood by many people. Seventy-seven per cent of the adults agreed with the statement that, 'making sure your bowels open every day is important for keeping healthy'. But those who agreed were not more likely to have reported constipation or to have taken laxatives or health salts than those who either felt neutral or disagreed with the statement. This was so even though older people agreed with the statement about a daily bowel movement more often than younger people. (Eighty-six per cent of those aged 65 or more agreed, 78% of those 35–64 and 68% of younger adults.) Older people also reported constipation more often. (Sixteen per cent of people aged 65 and over reported it, 8% of the younger adults.) They were also more likely to take laxatives. (See Table 59.) Men more often than women agreed that a daily bowel movement was important, 86% compared with 70%. But they were less likely to be constipated. Thirteen per cent of the women reported constipation during the two weeks asked about, 6% of the men. A higher proportion of women than men had taken laxatives or health salts, 20% compared with 14%.

Six per cent of the children had taken a laxative or health salts. The proportion was higher, 9%, among those under 5 than for those aged 5 or more, 4%. Sixty-nine per cent of parents of children agreed with the statement about a daily bowel movement. This proportion was similar to that of the adults aged 21 to 34. It seems that anxiety about frequent bowel movement has been declining over the years. Jefferys *et al.*[4] found that over a quarter of the children in their study had been given laxatives during a four-week period. Reid found that 22% of school entrants were given them at least once a week.[5] Both these studies were carried out during the nineteen-fifties. The present study found that only 3% of the children had been given laxatives during a two-week period.[6] So there seems to have been quite a dramatic decline during the past twenty years in the giving of laxatives to children.

For the indigestion remedies however there was no difference between the proportions of men and women who had taken them, and similar proportions of men and women reported having indigestion. Unlike analgesics and skin creams the taking of indigestion remedies increased with age. The trends with age for all the digestive system remedies are shown in Table 58. Nine per cent of the children had been given some kind of medicine for the digestive system, none of which had been prescribed.

[4] Jefferys, Margot, Brotherston, J. H. F. and Cartwright, Ann, 1960, 'Consumption of medicines on a working-class housing estate'.
[5] Reid, J. J. A., 1956, 'Regular use of laxatives by school-children'.
[6] This did not vary with social class, so the difference between the studies cannot be explained by the different class composition of the samples.

TABLE 58   *The consumption of remedies for the digestive system during a two-week period by adults in different age groups*

Percentage taking:	Age group							
	Chil-dren	21–24	25–34	35–44	45–54	55–64	65–74	75 and over
indigestion remedies (or gripe water)	3%	10%	6%	11%	13%	19%	24%	20%
laxatives	3%	4%	4%	6%	6%	9%	15%	26%
health salts	3%	9%	5%	6%	7%	8%	14%	16%
any of these	9%	17%	14%	19%	24%	31%	39%	44%
Number of people (= 100%)	519	81	230	289	269	258	194	87

Nineteen per cent of the babies had been given an indigestion remedy or gripe water, but only 1% of the other children.

Medicines for the respiratory system

Half the adults reported at least one respiratory symptom. 'Cough, catarrh or phlegm' were reported by more people than any other symptom apart from headache. Nearly a third of the sample reported these as having troubled them during the two weeks preceding the interview. Eighteen per cent had had a 'cold, flu, or running nose', 12% a sore throat and 15% reported breathlessness. The proportions of adults who reported the four respiratory symptoms asked about decreased, as expected, from the beginning of the field work in March to the end, in July. Thirty-one per cent of the adults interviewed during March reported 'colds, flu or running nose', 14% of those interviewed in July. The corresponding proportions for 'coughs, catarrh or phlegm' were 47% and 28%, for sore throat, 17% and 10%. 'Cough, catarrh or phlegm' was the only symptom asked about which was reported by proportionally more men than women. Thirty-five per cent of men reported them, 29% of women. One factor which contributes to this unusual difference in morbidity between the sexes is smoking. Sixty per cent of the men in the sample smoked cigarettes compared with 40% of the women; male smokers also smoked more on average than women. Smoking habits and the prevalence of respiratory symptoms are highly correlated as can be seen from Table 59. There were upward trends for both 'cough, catarrh or phlegm' and 'colds, flu or a running nose'; those smoking more reported more symptoms. There were no differences between men and women who smoked similar amounts. Many people recognised the ill-effects of their smoking. It was said to be the cause of 23% of 'coughs, catarrh and phlegm', 14% of the breathlessness and 7% of sore throats.

TABLE 59 *Reported incidence of cough, catarrh or phlegm and colds, flu or running nose among groups of people with different smoking habits*

	Proportions of people reporting	
	coughs, catarrh or phlegm	*colds, flu or running nose*
Non-smokers	24% (710)	16% (710)
1–4g. per day	37% (92)	18% (92)
5–14g. per day	38% (250)	18% (250)
15–24g. per day	41% (256)	24% (256)
25g.+ per day	51% (90)	24% (90)

1g. of tobacco is equal to 1 cigarette.

Figures in brackets refer to the number of adults on which the percentages were based (= 100%).

Thirteen per cent of the adults in the study had taken throat or cough remedies, 4% cold or congestion relievers. Three-tenths of these medicines were prescribed. Their consumption by smokers and non-smokers did not vary. Smokers were less likely to take medicines for their respiratory symptoms than non-smokers: 51% of the smokers' respiratory symptoms had been treated with medicine compared with 62% of the non-smokers' symptoms. Perhaps smokers, knowing that the habit contributes to the cause of their symptoms, are more fatalistic about them. They may feel that medicines can have little effect as long as they continue to smoke and so do not take them. They may even smoke an extra cigarette instead!

Twelve per cent of the children had taken cough or throat medicines, 3% cold and congestion relievers. There were no age or sex differences in the proportions of the children who had taken these medicines. There was however a clear trend with age in the proportion reported to have had 'coughs, catarrh or phlegm' and 'colds, flu or a running nose'. A quarter of the babies under two had these symptoms, and the proportion fell to a tenth of children aged 10–14. It seems that mothers were more cautious about treating younger children for these symptoms.

Tonics, vitamins and medicinal foods and drinks

Twelve per cent of the children had taken these kinds of medicines; 6% vitamins, 2% tonics and 4% medicinal foods. All three kinds were more likely to have been given to younger children. The trends are shown in Table 60. Only 6% of vitamins and tonics given to children were prescribed by a doctor. The use of some of them is however encouraged by child welfare services.

TABLE 60 *Proportions of children of different ages who had been given vitamins, medicinal foods and tonics, during a two-week period*

	Age group			
	under 2 years	2–4	5–9	10–14
Proportion who had been given:				
vitamins	16%	6%	4%	2%
medicinal foods	9%	5%	4%	1%
tonics	4%	4%	2%	1%
Number of children (= 100%)	68	113	169	169

Nearly a fifth of the adults had taken either a tonic, a vitamin preparation or a medicinal food or drink, including 'alcohol for medicinal purposes' during the two weeks. Five per cent had taken tonics, 6% vitamins, 4% medicinal foods and 4% alcohol. Women were twice as likely as men to have taken tonics and vitamins, though not medicinal foods or alcohol. There were no differences between the proportions of people in different age groups who had taken tonics or alcohol. But people under 55 were more likely to have taken vitamins than those aged 55 and over: 8% compared with 3%. The opposite was true for medicinal foods, 6% of the older age group having taken them compared with 3% of the younger.

Tonics and vitamins were taken relatively frequently by the adults: nineteen times on average during the two weeks. Many of them were taken for general health or preventive reasons or for tiredness. People who rated their health as poor or fair were more likely to take tonics than those who regarded it as excellent or good—8% compared with 3%.

It seems that many of these medicines are taken by people who develop a 'symbolic dependence' on them of the sort described by Joyce.[7] It is unlikely that the majority produce any physical improvement. As Bradshaw[8] says, 'most patent medicine tonics ... are of little or no value, quite apart from the lay person's difficulty in choosing the right one for his condition'. The same applies to vitamins which if taken in excess of the body's requirement are excreted very quickly. Vitamin deficiency is rare in this country and it would be difficult for a lay person to diagnose it precisely and decide which vitamins he needed even if he really did need them. Claims made for vitamins and the vitamin products have been so excessive that the Advertising Association[9] has told its members that it is doubtful whether any benefit at all can be derived by healthy persons taking vitamins in excess of their normal requirements as supplied by an adequate diet.

In fact 41% of the vitamins and 27% of the tonics taken by adults were prescribed, and 23·5 million prescriptions for tonics, iron and vitamins were dispensed from chemists in 1968: 9% of all prescriptions.[10] Many of these, as well as the self-prescribed ones, probably have a largely placebo effect. A recent study of vitamin B_{12},[11] which is only effective in treating pernicious anaemia, showed that the observed rate of prescribing for this was between three and twenty times greater than might be expected from the prevalence of pernicious anaemia. A third of the prescriptions had been written for conditions other than

[7] Joyce, C. R. B., 1968, 'Quantitative estimates of dependence on the symbolic function of drugs'.
[8] Bradshaw, S., 1966, *The Drugs You Take*, p. 131.
[9] Advertising Association, 1962, *Advertising of Vitamin Products*.
[10] Department of Health and Social Security, 1969, *Annual Report for 1968*, pp. 102–3.
[11] Cochrane, A. L., and Moore, F., 1971, 'Expected and observed values for the prescription of vitamin B_{12} in England and Wales'.

pernicious anaemia. More importantly, when the vitamin was prescribed for the disease it was often prescribed in greater quantities than necessary. It seems that not only do people buy for themselves substantial quantities of tonics and vitamins that can have no pharmacological efficacy but that doctors are also often prescribing them.

Drugs acting on the central nervous system

A tenth of the sample of adults had taken a sedative[12] drug during the two-week period, 1% an antidepressant, and another 1% some other type of drug acting on the central nervous system such as travel sickness tablets. The great majority, 94%, were obtained on a prescription. The number of prescriptions written for these drugs in National Health Service general practice has risen rapidly in recent years. In 1962[13] 27 million prescriptions were written for sedatives and anti-depressants, in 1968[14] the total was 42 million, a percentage increase of 56% compared with 32% for all other prescriptions. Part of this increase is no doubt due to the successful marketing of many new tranquillisers, especially non-barbiturates. Another factor may be a growth in community care; because these drugs are effective in controlling some forms of mental illness some patients no longer need to be in hospital and others can receive active treatment for conditions like depression which were once left untreated. The main reason given for taking sedatives was sleeplessness. Just over half the sedatives were taken for this but another 30% were taken for symptoms and ill-defined conditions such as 'nerves', 'depression' and 'to calm me down'. The rest, 16%, were for specific psychiatric conditions, for diseases of the nervous system like epilepsy or for other conditions such as a stroke.

People were asked at the interview whether they had experienced 'sleeplessness' or 'nerves, depression or irritability' during the previous two weeks.[15] Table 61 shows that far more women

---

[12] In this section the word 'sedative' is used as an abbreviation for 'sedatives, tranquillisers or sleeping tablets'.
[13] The Ministry of Health, 1963, *The Health and Welfare Services*: Report for 1962.
[14] Department of Health and Social Security, op. cit., pp. 102–3.
[15] Similar results have been found on other studies. See Silverman, C., 1968, *The Epidemiology of Depression*, p. 73.

than men reported these symptoms. It is therefore not surprising to find that more than twice as many women as men had taken sedatives in the two-week period: 13% compared with 6%.

TABLE 61　*Proportions of men and women reporting 'sleeplessness' and 'nerves, depression and irritability' and taking sedatives, sleeping tablets or tranquillisers*

	Men	Women
Proportion reporting sleeplessness	12%	20%
Proportion reporting nerves, depression or irritability	14%	27%
Proportion who had taken sedatives, sleeping tablets or tranquillisers	6%	13%
Number of adults (= 100%)	661	749

Age patterns were rather different. Sleeplessness increased with age but younger people more often reported 'nerves, depression and irritability' than older people. This can be seen from Table 62

TABLE 62　*Proportion of people in each age group reporting 'sleeplessness' and 'nerves, depression or irritability' and taking sedatives, sleeping tablets or tranquillisers*

	Age group						
	21–24	25–34	35–44	45–54	55–64	65–74	75+
Proportion reporting sleeplessness	11%	10%	12%	16%	22%	21%	23%
Proportion reporting nerves, depression or irritability	26%	26%	24%	22%	16%	13%	19%
Proportion who had taken sedatives, sleeping tablets or tranquillisers	1%	4%	7%	8%	14%	16%	23%
Number of adults (= 100%)	81	230	289	269	258	194	87

which also shows that the proportion taking sedatives followed the same age trend as sleeplessness but to a more marked degree. Although questions were not asked about people's views on

sleep it seems likely that the body's need for sleep is as mis-
understood as the need for a daily bowel movement was found
to be. People apparently need a diminishing period of sleep from
adolescence onwards. If people rate how well they sleep against
the norm of their youth then many people who find that they
cannot sleep for such long periods may feel that they suffer from
sleeplessness. This may partly explain the increase in the incidence
of sleeplessness and the taking of sedatives with age.[16] Unlike
other kinds of medicines the use of sedatives varied with social
class. More middle-class people, 12%, had taken them than
working class, 8%, but there were no class differences in the
proportion reporting 'sleeplessness' or 'nerves, depression or
irritability'.

Are middle-class people more likely to consult their doctor for
these nervous symptoms? If so this could explain why they were
more likely to take sedatives for them. We have no direct evidence
about this but answers to a hypothetical question suggest that
this is not the explanation. When people were asked what they
would do[17] about 'a constant feeling of depression for about
three weeks' and 'difficulty sleeping for about a week' working-
class people more often than middle-class thought they would
consult a doctor. (The figures for depression were 68% of the
middle class thinking they would consult a doctor compared
with 75% of the working class; and for sleeplessness 48% against
56%.) This suggests that the difference lies in the consulting
room. Once there middle-class patients may communicate their
demands and anxieties more effectively to the doctor or the
doctor may respond to their symptoms differently.

Sedatives and antidepressants had been taken by more people
in the survey than any other category of drug that is obtainable
only by prescription from a medical practitioner. Many of them
were taken regularly (two-thirds had been taken every day in the
two-week period) and many were taken over long periods, three-
fifths for more than a year. Earlier in this chapter we speculated
about the way in which people may become symbolically dependent on such medicines as tonics and vitamins that they take over

---

[16] Similar results were found on a study of doctors' prescribing habits. See Parish,
Peter A., 1971, 'The prescribing of psychotropic drugs in general practice'.
[17] 'Would you consult the doctor, do something yourself or what would you do—
or wouldn't you do anything?'

long periods. Psychotropic drugs may lead to physical dependence. They act on the central nervous system and some of them
may produce adverse reactions.

Another problem involved in the widespread use of these drugs
is their potential danger when taken by people who drive. A
survey[18] found that many drivers were unaware of the effect that
drugs could have on road behaviour. Most of these drivers were
not themselves taking drugs acting on the central nervous system.
The present survey suggests that even those people who are taking
these drugs are badly informed about their effects. People were
asked if anyone had told them whether their prescribed medicines
had any side effects or whether after taking them they should not
drink alcohol, drive a car, eat certain foods or take other drugs.
For only a fifth of the drugs acting on the central nervous system
did people recall having been told about any of these things.

Oral contraceptives

Forty-eight of the women in our sample had taken oral contraceptives during the two weeks before their interviews. This is 6·4
of the total sample of women over 21 years old and 10·7% of
those between 21 and 54. The highest proportion, 22%, of pill-
takers was found in the 25–34 age group. (See Table 63.) A survey

TABLE 63   *Percentage of women in each age group taking oral contraceptives*

	Age group			
	21–24	25–34	35–44	45–54
Proportion taking oral contraceptives	11%	21%	11%	1%
Number of women (= 100%)	47	123	141	138

of married women under 45 years old in 1967[19] found that for
17% the contraceptive pill was the method 'now' or 'last' used.
The comparable figure for married women under 45 in the present
study was 18%. The majority of women taking the pill, 70%,

[18] Automobile Association, 1969, 'The drugged driver'.
[19] Woolf, Myra, 1971, *Family Intentions*, p. 83.

had first had a prescription between one and five years before, only 2% earlier.

A recent study[20] of mothers who had just had a baby found that 57% of people taking contraceptive pills reported side effects. In the present study rather fewer, two-fifths, said that it caused side effects.[21] This is three times greater than for any other type of drug apart from the antibiotic, anti-infective group—a fifth of which were reported to cause side effects. Those taking oral contraceptives did not report appreciably more symptoms than women aged 21–54 not taking the pill, nor did they rate their health any differently, but they did report more headaches and 'nerves, depression and irritability'. Seventy-seven per cent of pill-takers reported headaches, compared with 54% of those not taking the pill; and 44% reported 'nerves, depression or irritability' compared with 30% of the others. This suggests that women taking the pill may be prone to these symptoms. They did not report either more or less of the other thirty symptoms we asked about.

Discussion

One of the more encouraging findings of this study in comparison with earlier inquiries is the dramatic decrease in laxative taking among children during the last ten to twenty years. We can only speculate about the reasons for this. Health education from health visitors and the mass media may have contributed both directly by discouraging the use of laxatives and indirectly over a longer period by altering habits of early pot training so that parents are less bowel oriented and concerned, even though many of them still believe that a daily bowel movement is important for keeping healthy.

The fact that undersirable habits like the regular dosing of children with laxatives do change may give encouragement to the health educators. One suggestion from this study may merit their attention. It seems plausible that at least part of the reason for the increase in reported sleeplessness with age is due to unrealistic expectations about their sleep among older people; and the relation between reported sleeplessness and sedative taking seems

20 Cartwright, Ann, 1970, *Parents and Family Planning Services*, p. 36.
21 'Do you think _____ has caused any symptoms or side effects? What?'

straightforward. If older people, particularly women, understood their sleep needs better, there might be less demand for sedatives.

There are other implications for health educators in the data about smoking and respiratory illnesses. Many smokers recognise that the habit causes such symptoms as cough, phlegm and bronchitis; but this understanding is not enough for them to give up smoking. They just never embark on, or they abandon, any attempt to relieve their symptoms with medicines. Such fatalism may make them immune to logical arguments about risks.

9

DISCUSSION

This report has presented data about medicine-taking habits from the point of view of both the consumer and the general practitioner as prescriber. In these conclusions we try to bring the main findings of the study together and to consider the implications. In doing this we draw on data from other surveys and venture rather further into interpretation and speculation than we have done in other chapters. The main points emphasised are the changing threshold at which illness is recognised, the efficacy of medication, the role of self-medication, the function of repeat prescribing and the differences in the doctor's and the patient's perception of the role of medical care.

Illness thresholds

One of the starting points for the study was the increase in both prescribed and non-prescribed medication in recent years. Other data suggested that there had been a change in the threshold level at which illness was translated into sickness absence[1] and it seemed likely that this had been accompanied by a change in the level at which medication was felt appropriate. These changes might occur on their own or they might stem from a more general lowering of the threshold at which illness is perceived at all. People's expectations about health may be rising and this may mean they are more likely to regard a headache or a corn as something wrong and to seek remedies for symptoms which were formerly accepted without any attempt at treatment.

Comparisons with another study in twelve areas of England and Wales done five years earlier support this.[2] The proportion of adults who thought they would consult their doctor about 'a

[1] Office of Health Economics, 1971, *Off Sick*, p. 16.
[2] Cartwright, Ann, 1967, *Patients and their Doctors*, pp. 36 and 107.

117

constant feeling of depression for about three weeks was 54% in the earlier study compared with 72% in the current one. And the proportions who would do so for 'difficulty in sleeping at night for about a week' were 45% and 53%. In addition the proportion of adults who said they thought their doctor would be a good person to talk to about a personal problem rose from 28% to 41%.

Yet there is no indication that general practitioner consultation rates are increasing. Possibly the accuracy of peoples' predictions about what they would do in different circumstances has changed. People may be more inclined to regard it as appropriate to consult their doctor about these conditions but no more likely to do so in practice. One reason for this might be that doctors had become more inaccessible—because of appointment systems, barriers created by receptionists and secretaries, and greater distances to travel. Another possibility is that, as more people feel that such symptoms as depression and sleeplessness and personal problems fall within the doctor's province, they are less likely to consult about more specifically physical symptoms than they did before. This might happen either because they themselves were now more aware of the psychological problems underlying their physical symptoms or because they now felt they could ask their doctor directly about their emotional problems.

The current study showed what sorts of symptoms people regarded as compatible with health. In fact two-thirds of the adults regarded their health as excellent or good but this same group reported an average of three symptoms present in the two weeks before they were interviewed. Complaints reported relatively frequently by the healthy were headaches, troubles with skin, teeth and feet and minor accidents. These were relatively common conditions and except for headaches they may be felt to be peripheral, affecting the person externally but not internally and therefore more easily discounted and not seen as basically threatening. They are conditions for which many remedies and reliefs are advertised and it seems likely that they are the sorts of symptoms for which medicines will increasingly be taken. No medicines had been taken for almost half the symptoms reported, so medicine taking may well continue to increase.

Discussion

The efficacy of medication

Just over half the adults had taken some medicine in the twenty-four hours before they were interviewed. Much of this medication was palliative and probably a great deal would be illogical or irrelevant in simple pharmacological terms. But the efficacy of medicine does not depend only on its pharmacological properties. The circumstances and manner in which it is prescribed, the relationship between patient and prescriber and the attitudes of the patient are all likely to contribute to its effectiveness.

Medicine taking fulfils other functions besides pharmacological ones. It may act as an indication that the person is sick and has assumed the sick role. It can show that the person is behaving appropriately in that role: he is trying to get better by taking medicine. In our positivistic society which tries to control its environment some form of action in adversity seems appropriate. To take no action seems fatalistic and weak. By taking medicine a person may feel he is asserting some control over the situation and of course a belief that he is hastening his recovery may be self-fulfilling.

Two-thirds of the medicines taken by adults were said to have helped their symptoms a lot. This is higher than might be expected from a simple placebo effect. An analysis of the placebo effect in a series of trials suggested that, rather constantly, about a third of people treated with placebos got satisfactory relief from them.[3]

So people felt most of the medicines they took were effective, and less than one in fifteen were said to have caused side effects. The benefit may be illusory in clinical terms; it could result from their expectations and optimism or be the specific effects of the drug, but it helped them. As for the 4% of medicines said not to have helped at all, people who took those may have been relieved from feelings of guilt for not having attempted to do something about their illnesses and feelings of remorse for not having tried something that could have helped. All these are possible benefits of medication and most apply to self-prescribed as well as to prescribed drugs. In fact the self-prescribed drugs were thought to have been at least as efficacious as the prescribed ones by the adults who had taken them.

[3] Beecher, H. K., 1955, 'The powerful placebo'.

119

Discussion

The role of self-medication

In a two-week period the ratio of self-prescribed to prescribed medicines taken by adults was roughly two to one, but within a twenty-four-hour period the ratio was nearer one to one as prescribed medicines were taken more frequently. Clearly taking non-prescribed medicines is a popular activity; two-thirds of the adults had done so in the two weeks before the interview. And only a small proportion, a tenth, of the non-prescribed medicines taken by adults had been first suggested by a doctor; most were the suggestions of parents, friends, neighbours, husbands or wives or other relatives. But must doctors not only regarded self-treatment as appropriate for many ailments, they also encouraged and advised their patients about how and when to do this. The relief of simple symptoms with relatively harmless remedies taken occasionally over short periods seems the appropriate role of self-medication. Possible dangers are mis-diagnosis and misuse. People may self-treat conditions which need medical intervention. The frequency of such 'errors' cannot be estimated from this study but the data suggest that adults tended to use self-medication as an alternative to medical consultation and some adults may turn to self-treatment when medical consultation has been found unsuccessful. Adults seemed less likely to consult about depression, persistent headaches and acute sore throats than doctors felt appropriate. For children self- or parent-medication seemed to be used more as a supplement to medical consultation. If conditions are self-treated before a doctor is seen this may make diagnosis more difficult for the doctor as self-prescribed medicines may mask more serious complaints.

Abuse of non-prescribed drugs is also difficult to define. A fifth of the self-prescribed medicines taken by adults in the two-week period had been taken every day during that time. Tonics and vitamins were the types of medicines most frequently involved. As these were often taken for general feelings of malaise rather than for more specific symptoms it may be that people were resorting to such self-treatment in circumstances when medical consultation would have been more appropriate and helpful. But most of the medicines that were taken frequently were prescribed ones.

Discussion

Function of repeat prescribing

About two-thirds of prescriptions were repeats, for the same drugs that people had before, and among the prescribed medicines that adults were currently taking half had been repeated five or more times and a fifth at least forty times. A quarter of the medicines first prescribed a year or more before the interview were drugs acting on the central nervous system, and one in twelve of the adults had been taking such drugs for a year or more. The widespread use and availability of such drugs has obvious implications in relation to drug dependence, suicide attempts, experimental use and abuse and also to driving and road safety. And it is the consumption of psychotropic drugs which has increased more rapidly than that of other types of drugs in recent years.

The doctors in the study seemed to underestimate the frequency of repeat prescribing. This is consistent with the 'shock and embarrassment' of doctors taking part in another study[4] when they discovered that a quarter of the patients they saw received a repeat prescription and very little else.

Balint and his colleagues have argued that long-term repeat prescribing suggests a failure of doctor–patient communications. The patient needs help: he has a continuing unsolved problem. It may be that the doctor can give him only palliative treatment, or that the doctor feels he needs to spend more time than he can spare to give more intensive care, or it may be a problem the doctor feels unsympathetic towards or one which he has not fully understood or diagnosed. In any of these ways long-term repeat prescribing may be symptomatic of an unsatisfactory relationship. But at least the relationship continues even if it is a rather tenuous one with little personal contact.

Role perception

Half the doctors thought that at least a quarter of their consultations were for conditions which people could treat themselves. In fact when the doctors were asked whether they felt it was appropriate for patients to consult them about a number of

[4] Balint, Michael; Hunt, John; Joyce, Dick; Marinker, Marshall and Woodcock, Jasper, 1970, *Treatment of Diagnosis*, pp. 133–5.

conditions they were far from unanimous in their views. Not surprisingly there was even less consensus among the patients. Unfortunately for doctor–patient relationships the views of individual patients and their particular doctors on this were unrelated.

This difference in role perception means that patients often do not consult about conditions which doctors could help or relieve. There is mounting evidence from other sources that this is particularly true for elderly patients. Many old people may accept their disabilities as an inevitability of old age and so will not consult a doctor until the symptoms are advanced or a crisis occurs.[5] Other studies have shown that people have not consulted about certain problems even though they have seen their doctor for other reasons.[6] 'To see a doctor about one condition does not necessarily mean he will ask or find out about other problems.'[7] Old people are probably particularly sensitive to feelings that they 'do not want to bother the doctor'. If doctors do not probe, or if they resent the 'while I'm here doctor' gambit which often precedes the introduction of another problem, patients will feel rationed to a single complaint at a consultation. Doctors will then be unaware of the multiple morbidity prevalent among many of their elderly patients.

The differences in role perception that exist between the doctors themselves stem from the lack of job definition in general practice. The differences between patients and doctors arise not only because patients do not feel it appropriate to consult about some things but also because they have unduly high expectations or hopes about the medical profession's ability to cure or relieve other conditions. In practice a continuing 'demand' of patients for help for the common tribulations of coughs, muscle and joint pains, backache and nervous disorders is surely appropriate. If doctors were consulted only about the diseases they could cure they would be less aware of common needs.

To sum up, medicine taking is a common activity, frequently indulged in, often over long periods. It serves a variety of needs, many of them social and psychological rather than purely pharma-

[5] Williamson, J., 1967, 'Detecting disease in clinical geriatrics'.
[6] Cartwright, Ann; Hockey, Lisbeth and Anderson, John L., *Life before Death* (in press).
[7] Lance, Hilary, 1971, 'Transport services in general practice', p. 46.

cological. The most powerful and harmful drugs can only be obtained on prescription and much prescribing is done on a repeat basis over long periods. Some of the demand for drugs probably arises because of inadequacies in the doctor–patient relationship, some is a reflection of the impotence of the medical profession and medical science to cure or relieve many common ailments.

THE SAMPLES OF AREAS, ADULTS, HOUSEHOLDS AND CHILDREN

Selection of areas

The study was carried out in fourteen parliamentary constituencies in England, Wales and Scotland. The 618 constituencies in England, Wales and Scotland were first divided into two groups: the wholly urban areas and those with some rural districts. They were then stratified by eleven economic regions: Northern, Yorkshire and Humberside, North West, East Midlands, West Midlands, East Anglia, South West, South East, Greater London Council, Wales and Monmouthshire and Scotland. Within each region the wholly urban constituencies were listed in order of the ratio of Conservative to Labour votes at the 1966 General Election and the partly rural in order of the percentage of electors living in rural districts. The number of electors in each constituency were listed cumulatively and the total for England and Wales divided by twelve to give the sampling interval. A number less than this was taken from a book of random numbers and the constituencies in which the number and subsequent additions of the sampling interval fell were taken as the study areas. A similar procedure was carried out to select two areas in Scotland.

The fourteen areas selected at random in this way were the wholly urban areas of Grimsby, Liverpool–Walton, Birmingham–Hall Green, Swansea–West, Woolwich–East, Merton & Morden, Southampton–Itchen and Glasgow–Shettleston; and the partly rural areas of Knutsford, Worcestershire–South, Dorset–West, New Forest, Canterbury and West Lothian. Some statistics about the areas are in Table A.

The sample of adults

One hundred and fifty people were drawn at random from each of the twelve Registers of Electors in England and Wales. As the population of Scotland is about one-tenth that of England and Wales only ninety people were chosen from each of the two Scottish areas. The final sample of 1,980 was made up of 1,800 in England and Wales and 180 in Scotland. Initially 69% of those adults still living in the study areas were interviewed. Because we felt this response rate was too low those people who were not contacted or who had refused were approached again. This increased the response rate to 76%. It

TABLE A *The fourteen study areas*

Areas	Economic Region	Conservative, Labour votes ratio 1970	Total Population 1966	Percentage living in rural districts 1966	Proportion of economically active males over 15 in non-manual occupations 1966 %	% in Registrar General's Social Class I and II in the sample
Merton and Morden	Greater London	1·2	64,570	—	50·4	25·0
Woolwich–East	Greater London	0·5	69,070	—	29·9	12·2
Swansea–West	Wales and Monmouthshire	0·9	85,760	—	38·9	24·8
Canterbury	South East	2·2	101,800	21·4	38·2	40·7
Liverpool–Walton	North West	0·8	79,080	—	26·2	7·4
Southampton–Itchen	South East	No Conservative candidate. M.P. was Speaker	112,320	—	29·2	16·8
Knutsford	North West	2·9	95,600	34·3	50·3	44·9
New Forest	South East	2·7	103,270	66·6	33·3	28·4
Grimsby	Yorkshire & Humberside	0·7	95,020	—	26·8	10·9
West Dorset	South West	2·0	66,190	55·3	34·5	37·6
Worcestershire–South	West Midlands	2·4	93,020	55·9	36·9	35·5
Birmingham–Hall Green	West Midlands	1·5	83,590	—	37·0	22·4
Glasgow–Shettleston	Scotland	0·4	67,190	—	19·6	5·3
West Lothian	Scotland	0·3	102,050	49·5	21·8	12·1

varied from 72% in the two London constituencies to 83% in Liverpool–Walton. Finally 1,412 adults were interviewed.

A comparison of the age and sex structure of the sample of adults interviewed with the population of England, Wales and Scotland is given in Table B. There were no differences between the proportions of men and

TABLE B   *Age and sex of sample of adults interviewed compared with population*

	Sample	Population of England, Wales and Scotland aged 21 and over [a]
	%	%
Sex		
Male	46·9	47·1
Female	53·1	52·9
	%	%
Age		
21–24	5·8	7·8
25–34	16·3	17·8
35–44	20·5	19·2
45–54	19·1	19·0
55–64	18·3	18·0
65–74	13·8	11·7
75+	6·2	6·5
Number of adults (= 100%)	1,412	35,334,32

[a] These distributions were obtained from the 1966 10% sample census data.

women but there were fewer people aged 21–24 in the sample and rather more aged 65–74 than expected. If the sample is reweighted to allow for this bias, the proportion who had taken prescribed medicines in the two weeks before interview rises from 41% to 45% and the proportion taking non-prescribed medicines remains unchanged.

The sample of households

The 969 households were chosen from the original sample of adults. For each person in the sample the number of names registered at the same address was noted. This number gives the relative probability of selection of that address. All the addresses where just one name was registered were taken, one in two of those with two names, one in three of those with three names, and so on. In Glasgow many of the addresses were occupied by large numbers of electors. Here the number of electors with the same surname as the sample adult was noted and this was used to determine the probability of selection. If this had not been done the sample of households in Glasgow would have been very small. The sample of households selected in this way has two limitations. First, households consisting only of people under the age of 21 are not included. Second, in England and Wales households at addresses containing more than one household will be under-represented since we only included the household in which our sample adult lived. In Glasgow households containing people with more than one surname will be over-represented. The effect of these biases does not appear to be great. Three per cent of the households in our sample excluding Glasgow said they lived at addresses where there was more than one household. Table C shows the

TABLE C *A comparison of the sample interviewed with the 1966 sample Census for household size*

Number of people in household	England and Wales		Scotland		England, Wales and Scotland	
	Sample	Census	Sample	Census	Sample	Census
	%	%	%	%	%	%
One	15	15	23	16	16	15
Two	29	30	24	27	29	30
Three	20	21	11	20	19	21
Four	20	18	20	18	20	18
Five	10	9	11	10	10	9
Six or more	6	7	11	9	6	7
Average number of persons per household	3·0	3·0	3·2	3·1	3·0	3·0
Number of households (= 100%)	607	15,359,68	62	1,600,88	669	16,960,56

distribution by household size for the sample who responded compared with England, Wales and Scotland. There were no significant differences. Altogether there were 969 households in our sample. For 686 (71%), information was obtained about the medicines in the home.

The sample of children

The sample of children included all children under 15 living in the sample of households. The number of children in the household was established for 874, 90%, of them.[1] Five hundred and ninety-one had no children, the other

[1] When the person in our sample was not prepared to answer our questions about medicines the interviewer still tried to find out if there were any children in the household.

TABLE D Number of households and children in each area

	Merton and Morden	Woolwich–East	Swansea–West	Canterbury	Liverpool–Walton	Southampton–Itchen	Knutsford	New Forest	Grimsby	West Dorset	Worcestershire–South	Birmingham–Hall Green	Glasgow–Shettleston	West Lothian	All areas
Size of sample of households	74	73	71	79	74	75	72	80	76	68	70	72	44	41	969
The number of households about which information obtained on medicines in the home	49	49	48	56	58	56	53	60	53	38	53	51	29	33	686
The number of households with children under 15 for which detailed information was obtained	18	19	17	21	23	26	11	22	24	10	26	14	14	12	257
The number of children for which information was obtained	33	37	33	45	45	52	21	42	52	19	51	25	36	28	519
Proportion of households at addresses with only one household	93%	96%	95%	94%	100%	98%	96%	100%	98%	100%	98%	100%	63%	97%	96%

283 had a total of 583 children under 15 years old. Information was obtained from parents for 519, 89%, of them. Table D gives the numbers of households and children in each area. Table E shows the age and sex of the sample of children. They did not differ significantly in these ways from the population.

TABLE E *Age and sex of sample of children compared with population*

	Sample	England, Wales and Scotland[a]
Sex of children under fifteen	%	%
Male	53·3	51·3
Female	46·7	48·7
Age	%	%
Under 2	13·1	14·9
2–4	21·7	21·8
5–9	32·6	33·0
10–14	32·6	30·3
Number of children under 15 (= 100%)	519	12,173,66

[a] These distributions were obtained from the 1966 10% sample census data.

Combination of results from adults and children

The results for adults and children are mainly presented separately in the report. They were selected in different ways and those aged 15–20 are not included in either sample. However, in looking at the study data on prescriptions some comparisons are made with national statistics which are based on prescriptions for all age groups. For this purpose prescriptions for our sample of adults and children have been added together even though we have no data for the intermediate age group. In 1968 people aged 15–20 made up 9% of the population. If they are omitted the proportion of children under 15 is 26% and of adults aged 21 or more 74%. When our sample of adults and children are added children account for 27% of the total, adults 73%.

THE SAMPLE OF GENERAL
PRACTITIONERS

This appendix discusses and attempts to evaluate various sources of bias in the sample of general practitioners. Possible bias derives from three sources: the way the areas were chosen, the way doctors were chosen within the areas, their response rate.

Areas

The areas were selected with probability proportional to the number of electors. Once this has been done equal weight should be attached to each of the areas to give a random sample.[1] This was done for the sample of adults by taking equal numbers in the twelve areas in England and Wales and equal numbers in the two Scottish areas. Because the sample of general practitioners was obtained through the adults and because the areas varied so much in population size (from 112,320 to 64,570) the number of doctors reported by people in the areas varied from 56 to 30. The result is that doctors from the

TABLE F   *Number of adults reporting the same doctor*

Number of adults with same doctor	Number of doctors	Number of adults
1	254	254
2	143	286
3	91	273
4	47	188
5	29	145
6	20	120
7	10	70
8 or more	4	38
Total	598	1,374

larger areas may be over-represented. One way to correct this bias is by weighting each doctor by the number of adults in the study who said he was their doctor, so that doctors mentioned by one person are included once, by two people twice, etc. The distribution is given in Table F. It shows, for

[1] A random sample means, statistically, that each unit has an equal chance of being selected.

Appendix II

example, that 20 doctors were each reported by 6 different people. These 20 doctors just appear once in the unweighted sample but are each given a weight of 6 in the weighted sample making a total of 120, because 120 people had these doctors.

TABLE G   *Comparison of selected doctors with weighted sample of adults' doctors*

(Data from the Department of Health and Social Security)

	Reported doctors	Adults' doctors (weighted sample)
Sex:	%	%
Men	93	94
Women	7	6
Age:	%	%
Under 35	9	8
35–44	32	31
45–54	30	34
55–64	22	21
65 and over	7	6
Number of doctors in practice:	%	%
One	21	20
Two	29	28
Three	26	27
Four	15	15
Five or more	9	10
Doctor eligible for rural practice payments:	%	%
Yes	26	27
No	74	73
Type of area:	%	%
Designated	27	27
Intermediate	17	17
Restricted	8	8
Open	48	48
Number on which percentages are based (= 100%)	583	1,354

Table G shows the effect of this reweighting on a number of characteristics for which information was obtained from the Department of Health and Social Security.[2] The first column shows the distribution among the *reported*

[2] Fifteen (3%) of the 598 doctors reported by adults could not be traced in the Department of Health and Social Security records, mainly because people gave inadequate information, or the doctor was found to have died, retired or moved.

Appendix II

doctors (each doctor being included once irrespective of the number of his patients in the sample of adults), and the second column the distribution among the *adults' doctors* with doctors reweighted according to the number of their patients in the sample. There are no significant differences with these variables. The unweighted sample of reported doctors has generally been used in the report for analyses which involve doctors only. Cross analyses of adults' and doctors' characteristics are of course based on the weighted sample.

Selection within areas

The general practitioners are the doctors of a randomly selected sample of adults. This has several implications:

1 The same doctor was reported by more than one of the adults in the study. This bias can be corrected by weighting, but in practice, as has been shown, this makes little difference.

2 Doctors who work only with children will be under-represented or missing.

3 Doctors with large numbers of patients will have a greater chance of being included than doctors with small numbers since the chance of being included is related to the number of adults over 21 years old among their patients. No estimate of the extent of this bias was possible, but it is in many ways a reasonable one.

Response

Less than 1% of the adults did not have a doctor. Two per cent did not give us enough information for us to trace him. The remaining 1,374 told us about 598 doctors. Four of those are known to have died, ten had retired or moved and three questionnaires were returned by the post office, the name and address untraced. Of the remaining 581, 326 completed and returned the questionnaire, a response rate of 56%. Altogether we have information about the doctors of 54% of the adults interviewed. This response rate is low. Variations in the response rate with some characteristics of the doctors and their practices obtained from the Department of Health and Social Security are given in Table H. Younger doctors were more likely to reply than older doctors. Sixty-two per cent of those under 50 replied, 47% of those aged 50 or more. Doctors practising in intermediate and restricted areas were more likely to reply than those living in either designated or open areas where list sizes are likely to be larger. The sex of the doctor, number of doctors in the practice, eligibility for rural practice payments and differences in any of the prescribing costs were not related to response.

There was some suggestion from the information given by the adults that general practitioners who did not collaborate differed in some ways from those who did. Some comparisons are shown in Table I. Eighty-five per cent of the adults' doctors who completed the questionnaire were thought to have enough time to listen and do everything necessary for patients, fewer of those people's doctors who did not reply, 76%, were felt to have enough time. This suggests that the doctors who did not collaborate were busier than the others and that one reason for non-collaboration was lack of time. Adults were also asked whether they would discuss a personal problem with

TABLE H   *Variation in response with some characteristics of doctors*

	Proportion completed questionnaire	Number of doctors (= 100%)
Sex:		
Male	56%	541
Female	56%	42
Age:		
under 35	58%	52
35–39	62%	76
40–44	64%	111
45–49	61%	89
50–54	45%	88
55–59	47%	76
60–64	55%	53
65 and over	39%	38
Number of doctors in practice:		
One	48%	121
Two	56%	167
Three	59%	151
Four	60%	89
Five or more	53%	55
Doctor eligible for rural practice payments:		
Yes	57%	154
No	55%	429
Type of area:		
Designated	52%	155
Open	53%	279
Intermediate	62%	101
Restricted	63%	48

their doctor. Forty-four per cent of those whose doctors replied said they would, 37% of the others. This may also reflect a lack of time on the part of the doctor. However, the patients of those doctors who did not collaborate had consulted their doctors a similar number of times during the previous year to those people whose doctors completed the questionnaire. More importantly for the study, there were no differences in the proportions of people who had taken medicine, either prescribed or non-prescribed.

TABLE I *Some comparison of adults whose doctors collaborated in the study with those whose doctors did not*

	Adults whose general practitioner collaborated in study	Adults whose general practitioner did not collaborate in study
Proportion who had taken:	%	%
any medicine	81	80
prescribed medicine	42	40
non-prescribed medicine	69	66
Number of consultations during the previous twelve months:	%	%
none	27	28
one	22	20
2–4	29	30
5–9	10	10
10 or more	12	12
Doctor thought to have enough time to listen and do all that is necessary:	%	%
Yes	85	76
No	15	24
Person thought he would discuss a personal problem with his doctor:	%	%
Yes	44	37
No	52	55
Uncertain	4	8
'Reliance on the doctor score':	%	%
score } low (0–3)	54	56
high (4–6)	46	44
'Reliance on self-treatment score':	%	%
low (0 or 1)	45	44
score { (2)	31	30
high (3–6)	24	26
Number of adults (= 100%)	763	611

Appendix II

Prescribing patterns

Up to now we have been describing the effect, or lack of effect, of the various possible sources of bias on fairly general and basic characteristics of the general practitioners and their types of practice. What about their

TABLE J *Comparison of selected doctors with weighted sample of adults' doctors*
(Prescribing data from the Department of Health and Social Security.)

	Reported doctors	Adults' doctors (weighted sample)
Numbers of prescriptions per person on doctors' list:	%	%
Less than $(\bar{x} - 2\sigma)$	15	15
$(\bar{x} - 2\sigma)$ but less than $(\bar{x} - \sigma)$	34	34
$(\bar{x} - \sigma)$ but less than $\bar{x}$	33	33
$\bar{x}$ but less than $(\bar{x} + \sigma)$	13	14
$(\bar{x} + \sigma)$ but less than $(\bar{x} + 2\sigma)$	3	3
$(\bar{x} + 2\sigma)$ or more	2	1
Average cost per prescription:	%	%
Less than $(\bar{x} - 2\sigma)$	2	1
$(\bar{x} - 2\sigma)$ but less than $(\bar{x} - \sigma)$	16	17
$(\bar{x} - \sigma)$ but less than $\bar{x}$	36	39
$\bar{x}$ but less than $(\bar{x} + \sigma)$	31	30
$(\bar{x} + \sigma)$ but less than $(\bar{x} + 2\sigma)$	11	10
$(\bar{x} + 2\sigma)$ or more	4	3
Average cost per person on doctors' list:	%	%
Less than $(\bar{x} - 2\sigma)$	3	3
$(\bar{x} - 2\sigma)$ but less than $(\bar{x} - \sigma)$	10	10
$(\bar{x} - \sigma)$ but less than $\bar{x}$	38	36
$\bar{x}$ but less than $(\bar{x} + \sigma)$	38	40
$(\bar{x} + \sigma)$ but less than $(\bar{x} + 2\sigma)$	8	9
$(\bar{x} + 2\sigma)$ or more	3	2
Number on which percentages are based ($= 100\%$)	564	1,317

$\bar{x}$ represents mean
σ represents standard deviation

prescribing patterns? The Department of Health and Social Security also provided some information on the prescribing costs of the doctors.[3] These were: number of prescriptions per person on doctors' list, average cost per prescription, average cost per person on doctors' list and the month and year when the analysis was made. These figures are collected from E.C.10

[3] Thirty-four (6 per cent) of the doctors could not be traced in these records.

prescription forms for each doctor during one month of each year. As the prescribing by the doctors in the study had been analysed in ten different months from March 1969 to March 1970 the absolute figures could not be used as prescribing varies so much from season to season. Instead, prescribing in each month was considered separately.

TABLE K   *Comparison of the prescribing data of doctors who did and those who did not respond to the postal questionnaire*

	Doctors who:	
	responded	failed to respond
Numbers of prescriptions per person on doctors' list	%	%
Less than $(\bar{x} - 2\sigma)$	16	14
$(\bar{x} - 2\sigma)$ but less than $(\bar{x} - \sigma)$	34	35
$(\bar{x} - \sigma)$ but less than $\bar{x}$	31	34
$\bar{x}$ but less than $(\bar{x} + \sigma)$	15	11
$(\bar{x} + \sigma)$ but less than $(\bar{x} + 2\sigma)$	3	4
$(\bar{x} + 2\sigma)$ or more	1	2
Average cost per prescription:	%	%
Less than $(\bar{x} - 2\sigma)$	2	2
$(\bar{x} - 2\sigma)$ but less than $(\bar{x} - \sigma)$	13	20
$(\bar{x} - \sigma)$ but less than $\bar{x}$	38	33
$\bar{x}$ but less than $(\bar{x} + \sigma)$	32	30
$(\bar{x} + \sigma)$ but less than $(\bar{x} + 2\sigma)$	11	12
$(\bar{x} + 2\sigma)$ or more	4	3
Average cost per person on doctors' list:	%	%
Less than $(\bar{x} - 2\sigma)$	3	3
$(\bar{x} - 2\sigma)$ but less than $(\bar{x} - \sigma)$	12	9
$(\bar{x} - \sigma)$ but less than $\bar{x}$	36	39
$\bar{x}$ but less than $(\bar{x} + \sigma)$	37	40
$(\bar{x} + \sigma)$ but less than $(\bar{x} + 2\sigma)$	10	6
$(\bar{x} + 2\sigma)$ or more	2	3
Number of doctors (= 100%)	319	245

X represents mean
σ represents standard deviation

For each of the ten months the means and standard deviations of the three different costs were calculated, thirty means in all. The numbers on which these means were based varied from 9 to 164; the number of doctors in the sample whose prescribing had been assessed during the same month. For three of the months there were only nine doctors in the sample whose prescribing had been assessed, a total of twenty-seven doctors, 5% of the sample.

Codes were drawn up using one standard deviation as the difference between each coding value. This made it appropriate to compare data from all the doctors whenever their prescribing was studied. Table J shows the effect on these three prescribing averages of correcting for the way the doctors were selected. The reweighting had no significant effect. Prescribing rates and costs were also unrelated to response rates. This is shown in Table K.

Summary

Although there are three sources of bias affecting the sample of general practitioners who completed and returned the postal questionnaire only one important discrepancy has emerged. This is related to the very low response rate of 56%. Younger doctors were more likely to reply and are therefore over-represented in the sample. But in spite of the low response the sample seems reasonably representative in relation to prescribing patterns.

APPENDIX III

COMPARISON OF THE TWO
CLASSIFICATIONS OF MEDICINES

The medicines were classified in two ways: first by the way people described them in response to our check list,[1] secondly in a more pharmacological way by the body system on which they are reputed to act and within each system by the reputed effect of the medicine. This classification was more comprehensive than the check list because it had categories for drugs like antibiotics and cardio-vascular and genito-urinary preparations.

The two systems differ in other ways. Some of the check-list categories were combined in the pharmacological classification, for example: *Gargles, mouthwashes* and *throat lozenges or sweets* were grouped together under 'mouth and throat preparations', (04) *health salts* were combined with *laxatives* (08) since they are primarily laxative in effect, *corn pads* were included with *dressings* (07) and *foot powders or ointments* with the appropriate skin category, *medicinal foods* were included in a single category with *alcohol and other drink used medicinally* (79). Other check-list groups were divided up, for example: *cough medicines* were separated from *throat lozenges* and put in a group with other lower respiratory medicines taken internally (05), *cold and congestion relievers* were divided into those acting locally on the nose (2X) and those acting systemically (2Y), *skin ointments* were divided between five categories: (a) those with a primarily soothing, emollient or irritation relieving effect (02), (b) those with a reputed therapeutic action such as anti-infective, keratolytic or antiseptic action (49), (c) preventive items such as barrier creams, insect repellants and suntan lotions (40), (d) other local preparations such as general antiseptics, germicides, disinfectants and cleaners (4X), and finally, (e) cortico-steroid skin preparations (4Y). Some problems arose because people did not always know what medicines they were taking or they did not know their intention.

Twenty-two per cent of the sample of adults had, during the last two weeks, taken a medicine which they put in the 'other' category on the interview check list. Forty per cent of these medicines had to be coded as inadequate on the pharmacological classification, another 22% could be regarded as genuine 'other' medicines not on the check list e.g. anti-rheumatics, anti-biotics and cardio-vascular and genito-urinary preparations. The rest, i.e. 38%, could have been fitted into the check-list categories but were not. This may have been because the respondent knew the proper name of the drug but did not know its action in lay terms. This posed a problem in isolating

[1] See Table 13, Chapter 3.

those people who had taken, for example, a pain-killer. We could isolate those people who *said* they had taken at least one at the check list during the interview. But we knew from our analyses of the medicines that people put into the 'other' category that there were eight more pain-killers taken by people who had not acknowledged the fact. This suggests that the proportion of people who had taken a pain-killer during the two-week period, 40·8%, (see Table 13 in Chapter 3) is an underestimate by a maximum 0·6% assuming that the eight pain-killers were taken by eight different people. (Without looking at the punched cards which represent those eight pain-killers we cannot know how many people are involved as some people were taking more than one brand.) However, fifteen of the medicines thought by respondents to be pain-killers were not, which means that the percentage of people taking pain-killers, now estimated at 41·4% is an overestimate by 1·1% reducing the proportion to 40·3%. The position then is that 40·8% of the sample said they had taken aspirin or another pain-killer when presented with a check list of medicines at an interview. Taking account of how these analgesic medicines and those medicines in the 'other' category were coded pharmacologically (with the Jasper Woodcock classification) we have reduced the estimate to 40·3%. Further problems arise because some of the 'cold relievers' people had taken were in fact analgesics which if added would raise the proportion to 41·6%.

As can be appreciated it was impractical to continue in this way to get an exact proportion of people who had taken any one kind of medicine asked about on the check list. The same procedure was carried out to estimate the proportion of people who had taken sedatives, sleeping tablets or tranquillisers. The corrections altered the proportion by 0·2%.

In fact many of the estimates of the proportions taking different medicines are likely to be under-estimates because of the large proportion, 25%, of prescribed medicines that we could not include in the pharmacological classification because people were not able to give us enough information about them.

APPENDIX IV

VARIATIONS BETWEEN AREAS
AND DIFFERENT TIMES OF THE YEAR

It was impractical to do many analyses between the fourteen study areas in
this inquiry because of the timing of the interviews. The main bulk of the
interviewing was carried out over four months from mid-March to mid-July,
and the areas were completed two at a time so there was no seasonal distribution of data within the areas. The mean number of medicines taken by the
adults fell from 2·7 in March to 1·8 in July.

To compare areas north and south of a line drawn between Bristol and
the Wash we looked at the eight areas where field work was done in April,
May and June. These were Canterbury, Southampton, New Forest and West
Dorset in the south and Swansea, Liverpool, Knutsford and Grimsby in the
north. In addition, Glasgow and West Lothian in Scotland were compared
with South Worcester and Birmingham in the Midlands. Field work in those
areas was done during June and July. This limited comparison between areas
in the north and south and between Scotland and the Midlands revealed no
significant differences in the numbers of medicines taken by adults.

Comparison between urban and partly rural areas is complicated by seasonal differences because more of the urban than the rural interviews were
done in the early part of the period. Comparisons within the early and later
times of the year again revealed no differences. In the report the only area
or north/south or urban/rural comparisons made are for factors which are
relatively unlikely to be affected by season such as the number of medicines
in people's homes. The prescribing habits of doctors were compared in ways
which took account of seasonal variations. Fortunately similar proportions
of people in the various social classes were interviewed in the different
months.

SCORES

Faith in doctors

This score was derived from a question to adults which asked, 'There are some things that doctors can cure completely, others that they can make feel better and some they can do very little about. Do you think they can generally cure, help or not help: rheumatism, a bad cold, corns, skin cancer, arthritis, depression, sleeplessness, frequent headaches, bronchitis?' The answers are in Table 36 in Chapter 5. A score for each person was calculated by counting two points for each 'cure' and one for each 'help' and dividing the total by the number of answers (excluding don't knows and inadequate answers). If the number of adequate answers was less than seven the score was coded as inadequate. The proportions of adults with different 'faith in doctors' scores are shown at Table L.

TABLE L   *Proportions of adults with varying 'faith in doctors' scores*

	Proportion of adults
Score:	%
0 but less than 0·4	1
0·4 but less than 0·7	6
0·7 but less than 1·0	19
1·0 but less than 1·3	47
1·3 but less than 1·6	24
1·6 but less than 1·9	3
1·9 or more	—
Number of adults (= 100%)	1,242

Neuroticism and extraversion

Two dimensions of human personality: extraversion–introversion and neuroticism–stability were measured with a twelve-item scale devised by S. B. G. and H. J. Eysenck.[1] Each adult and parent was asked as part of the interview:

[1] Eysenck, S. B. G. and Eysenck, H. J., 1964, 'An improved short questionnaire for the measurement of extraversion and neuroticism'.

Appendix V

'Here is a series of twelve questions. Would you please answer, yes or no, and try not to think too long about the exact meaning of them.'[2]

(a) Do you like plenty of excitement and bustle around you?
(b) Does your mood often go up and down?
(c) Are you rather lively?
(d) Do you ever feel 'just miserable' for no good reason?
(e) Do you like mixing with people?
(f) When you get annoyed do you need someone friendly to talk to about it?
(g) Would you call yourself happy-go-lucky?
(h) Are you often troubled about feelings of guilt?
(i) Can you usually let yourself go and enjoy yourself a lot at a gay party?
(j) Would you call yourself tense or 'highly strung'?
(k) Do you like practical jokes?
(l) Do you suffer from sleeplessness?

The extraversion score was calculated for each person by adding the number of 'yes' answers to questions (a), (c), (e), (g), (i), (k). The number of 'yes' answers to the other questions, i.e. (b), (d), (f), (h), (j), (l) made up the

TABLE M *Proportions of adults with different extraversion and neuroticism scores*

	Extraversion	Neuroticism
Score:	%	%
none	3	17
one	6	23
two	14	23
three	16	18
four	22	13
five	22	5
six	17	1
Mean score	3·8	2·1
Numbers of adults (= 100%)	1,387	1,387

person's neuroticism score. The proportion of adults with different extraversion and neuroticism scores are shown in Table M. The mean scores were 3·8 for extraversion and 2·1 for neuroticism. Eysencks' values for normal adults were 3·8 and 2·3.

[2] When they had answered the questions the interviewer explained: 'Those are the only questions like that. Please think carefully about the rest of the questions I'd like to ask you.'

Appendix V

Neuroticism, extraversion and smoking

There has been some discussion about the relationship between neuroticism and smoking recently. Eastwood and Trevelyan[3] found no evidence to support the hypothesis that smokers tend to be more neurotic than non-smokers. A study by Waters[4] in South Wales suggested that women smokers were more neurotic than women who did not smoke and there was a statistically significant correlation between the numbers of cigarettes smoked per day and the neurotic grade. This did not hold for men. Similarly, our data showed no relationship between smoking habits and the neuroticism score for men but an association for women. Twenty-nine per cent of women with a neuroticism score of none were smokers. This proportion rose to 55% of women with a score of six. There was also a suggestion that neuroticism increased with the amount smoked. Non-smoking women had a mean neuroticism score of 2·2, those smoking 1–4 a day a score of 2·5 and those smoking 5 or more 2·7. This supports the findings of the study carried out by Waters in South Wales.

Introversion–extraversion was related to smoking for both men and women. This has been shown before.[5] Average extraversion scores were 4·2 for male smokers and 3·7 for men who did not smoke; comparable figures for women were 3·8 and 3·5.

3 Eastwood, M. R. and Trevelyan, M. H., 1971, 'Smoking and neurotic illness'.
4 Waters, W. E., 1971, 'Smoking and neuroticism'.
5 Eysenck, H. J., 1965, *Smoking, Health and Personality*, p. 101.

APPENDIX VI

STATISTICAL SIGNIFICANCE

Chi-square, chi-square trend tests, tests on the difference between two proportions, correlation coefficients and t-tests have been applied constantly when looking at the data from this survey. They have influenced decisions about what differences to present and how much verbal 'weight' to attach to them. In general, attention has not been drawn to any difference which statistical tests suggest might have occurred by chance five or more times in 100.

TABLE N *Sampling errors*

	Value in total sample	Range in fourteen study areas	Sampling error	Estimated random sampling error[a]	Range ± two sampling errors
	%	%	%	%	%
Proportion of adults with no consultations in previous 12 months	27·8	20–35	1·2	1·2	25·4–30·2
Proportion with a 'high' neuroticism score of 4, 5 or 6	18·9	11–26	1·5	1·1	15·9–21·9
Proportion agreeing 'it is only sensible to take aspirin or something like that whenever you get a headache'	60·0	53–69	1·4	1·3	57·2–62·8
Proportion of adults taking prescribed medicines in two weeks before interview	41·3	31–48	1·4	1·3	38·5–44·1
Proportion taking indigestion remedies	14·4	9–20	1·0	0·9	12·4–16·4
Proportion in Social Classes IV and V	22·6	11–47	2·4	1·1	17·8–27·4

[a] If a random sample of the country, that is: $\sqrt{\dfrac{p \cdot q}{n}}$

Appendix VI

A difficulty which arises when presenting results from a study like this with nearly 500 items of basic information is that of selection. Inevitably not all cross-analyses are carried out—only about 1,200—and only a fraction of these are presented, which of course gives rise to difficulty in interpreting significance. Positive results are more often shown than negative ones. Readers may sometimes wonder why certain further analyses are not reported. Often, but not always, the analysis will have been done but the result found to be negative or inconclusive.

Table N shows the sampling errors for a number of characteristics in the sample of adults.[1] In general the sampling error is of the same order as the estimated random sampling error if the sample had been a straight one over the whole country and not just in fourteen areas. But the sampling error for social class is much larger than the estimated random sampling error because of the wide variations in this between areas.

[1] For the formula see Gray, P. G. and Corlett, T., 1950, 'Sampling for the Social Survey'.

CLASSIFICATION OF SOCIAL CLASS

Interview schedules for adults

The classification used is based on the Registrar-General's Classification of Occupations (1966).[1] This distinguishes five 'social classes':

I Professional, etc. occupations   IV Partly skilled occupations
II Intermediate occupations   V Unskilled occupations
III Skilled occupations

These classes are intended to reflect 'the general standing within the community of the occupations concerned'. Occupations in Classes II, III and IV are also classified as 'manual', 'non-manual' or 'agriculture'. In the analyses here the five classes are used, but Class III, skilled occupations, is divided into manual and non-manual groups to give a six-point scale. In a number

TABLE O   *Social class of sample adults compared with population*

	Sample	Population of Great Britain aged 21 and over[a]
	%	%
Middle class:		
I Professional	5	4
II Intermediate	20	17
III Skilled non-manual	14 ⎫	
	⎬ 53	48
Working class		
III Skilled manual	39 ⎭	
IV Semi-skilled	16	23
V Unskilled	6	8
Number of adults (= 100%)	1,325 [b]	35,203,56

[a] From Sample Census 1966, Economic activity, Tables, Part III.
[b] The 87 adults for whom inadequate information was obtained or who were students or members of the armed forces have been excluded.

---

[1] General Register Office, 1966, *Classification of Occupations.*

of instances the differences that emerge are between what can be described as the 'middle class' and 'working class', the former being most of the non-manual occupations (the Registrar-General's social classes I, II and III non-manual) and the latter almost entirely manual (III manual, IV and V). Table O shows the proportions of adults in these groups compared with the population of Great Britain. Men and single women were classified on the basis of their present occupations or their main occupations if retired. Married and widowed women were classified according to their husbands' present, last or main occupations. The children were classified by the social class of the sample adult living in the same household, who was interviewed.

The sample had fewer people in Social Classes IV and V than expected, even taking into account the wide variations in class distribution between areas. Reweighting to correct for this bias again had no significant effect even on characteristics related to class such as the average number of symptoms reported or the proportion taking sedatives.

THE QUESTIONNAIRES

Interview schedules for adults

HEALTH & MEDICINES
SURVEY

Questionnaire 1

I am from a social research organisation, the Medical Care Research Unit of the Institute of Community Studies.[1] I believe you have had a letter from us. We are doing a study about people's health and the medicines they take and we hope to write a report about it. I would like to ask you some questions. Anything you tell us will be treated as confidential and no one's name will be mentioned. We got your name from the electoral register.

Informant remembered receiving
  letter 1
Informant did not remember it 2

IF (2) GIVE INFORMANT ANOTHER
LETTER

1. During the last two weeks—
would you say your health has
been excellent, good, fair or
poor?
    Excellent 1
    Good 2
    Fair 3
    Poor................................... 4
    O.K. 5
Why do you think that?

2. Do you talk about health and
illness with your family and
friends a great deal, fairly often,
only occasionally or never?
    A great deal 6
    Fairly often.......................... 7
    Only occasionally 8
    Never................................. 9
    (Don't know)....................... Y

---

[1] This Medical Care Research Unit is now the Institute for Social Studies in Medical Care.

3. Do you read articles about
health and medicines in
newspapers or magazines:

PROMPT
⎰ Frequently 1
⎱ Occasionally 2
⎰ or hardly ever.............. 3
(never)........................ 4
(Don't know).............. 5

If 1 or 2 or 3 Have you read any
in the last two weeks?

Yes 6
No 7

If YES (6) What were they
about?

4. Do you have any books or
pamphlets on health and first aid
in your home that you refer to
when someone is not well?

Yes 1
No 2

If YES (1)
What are they?

5. I am going to read you two
descriptions of different kinds of
people. Which one sounds most
like you?

The first one is:

(a) Doctors don't know
everything about you, so I don't
always do exactly what they
advise.

The second one is:

(b) I always try to do exactly what
the doctor advises, even if it is
not very pleasant or easy.

Most like (a) 1
Most like (b) 2

6. Who is your own doctor?
RECORD NAME, INITIALS AND
ADDRESS

7. Is that under the National Health
Service or privately?

NHS 3
Privately 4

8. How long have you had this
particular doctor?

Less than a year..................... 1
1 year < 2 years 2
2 years < 5 years 3
5 years < 10 years................. 4
10 years < 15 years 5
15 years < 20 years 6
20 years or more 7

If less than a Year (1)
(a) Why did you change doctors?

Subject moved 1
Doctor retired, moved, died 2
Dissatisfied with old doctor...... 3
Other (specify) 4

If dissatisfied (3)
Why was that?

Continued overleaf

149

9. During the last 24 hours, that is since this time yesterday, have you taken or used any of these sorts of medicines? *For each one if no* what about in the last two weeks?					Type/ No.	What was it? Has it a brand name? What's in it? Have you taken any other (*category*) in the last two weeks? ENTER IN SEPARATE ROW	What was it for? *Probe to get symptom or condition/if contraceptive pill.* Was that as a contraceptive or for some other reason?	Did you it on a doctor's prescription?	
What about:	24 hrs Yes	No	2 wks Yes	No				Yes	N
					A				
1. Gargles or mouthwashes	1	0	1	0					
2. Health salts	2	0	2	0				1	
3. Indigestion remedies	3	0	3	0					
4. Laxatives	4	0	4	0					
5. Suppositories	5	0	5	0	B				
6. Throat or cough medicines or sweets	6	0	6	0					
7. Cold or congestion relievers	7	0	7	0				1	
8. Aspirin or other pain-killers	8	0	8	0					
9. Sedatives, sleeping tablets and tranquillisers	1	0	1	0					
10. Antidepressives, stimulants, pep pills	2	0	2	0	C				
11. Skin ointments or antiseptics	3	0	3	0				1	
12. Eye drops, lotions or ointments	4	0	4	0					
13. Embrocation or ointment to rub in	5	0	5	0					
14. Inhalants, drops or things to sniff up your nose	6	0	6	0	D				
15. Diarrhoea remedies	7	0	7	0					
16. Corn pads or foot powders, creams or dressings	8	0	8	0				1	
17. Tonics, rejuvenators	9	0	9	0					
18. Slimming aids	1	0	1	0					
19. Vitamin tablets	2	0	2	0	E				
20. Medicinal foods	3	0	3	0					
21. Surgical clothing, trusses, bandages, elastic stockings	4	0	4	0				1	
22. Alcohol—for medicinal purposes	5	0	5	0					
23. Hormones (or contraceptive pills)	6	0	6	0					
24. Travel or other kind of sickness pills	7	0	7	0	F				
25. Is there any other medicine, pills, ointments or injections you have had, either things the doctor prescribed or things you got yourself?	8	0	8	0				1	
Check So in the last two weeks you have taken or used _____ *Enter first type of medicine in table and ask questions across*					G				
								1	

If not prescribed en did you t take/use ___?	Who or what first gave you the idea?	*If taken in last 24 hrs* Do you take/use it every day?		How many times have you taken/used ___ in last 2 weeks?	Does this medicine help your (symptom): a lot, some or not at all?	Do you think ___ has caused any symptoms or side effects? *If Yes (3) What?*	
		Yes	No			Yes	No
than 2 wks......1 s < 1 mth ......2 h < 6 mths ......3 hs < 1 yr ....4 < 5 yrs............5 < 10 yrs ....6 rs or more 7		3	4	1..............1 2..............2 3, 4 ....3 5–9............4 10–14.........5 15–24.........6 25–29.........7 30–39.........8 40+...........9	a lot ....1 some ....2 not at all ....3 (uncertain) 4	3	4
than 2 wks......1 s < 1 mth ......2 h < 6 mths ......3 hs < 1 yr ....4 < 5 yrs............5 < 10 yrs ....6 rs or more 7		3	4	1..............1 2..............2 3, 4 ....3 5–9............4 10–14.........5 15–24.........6 25–29.........7 30–39.........8 40+...........9	a lot ....1 some ....2 not at all ....3 (uncertain) 4	3	4
than 2 wks......1 s < 1 mth ......2 h < 6 mths ......3 hs < 1 yr ....4 < 5 yrs............5 < 10 yrs ....6 rs or more 7		3	4	1..............1 2..............2 3, 4 ....3 5–9............4 10–14.........5 15–24.........6 25–29.........7 30–39.........8 40+...........9	a lot ....1 some ....2 not at all ....3 (uncertain) 4	3	4
than 2 wks......1 s < 1 mth ......2 h < 6 mths ......3 hs < 1 yr ....4 < 5 yrs............5 < 10 yrs ....6 s or more 7		3	4	1..............1 2..............2 3, 4 ....3 5–9............4 10–14.........5 15–24.........6 25–29.........7 30–39.........8 40+...........9	a lot ....1 some ....2 not at all ....3 (uncertain) 4	3	4
than 2 wks......1 s < 1 mth ......2 h < 6 mths ......3 hs < 1 yr ....4 < 5 yrs............5 < 10 yrs ....6 s or more 7		3	4	1..............1 2..............2 3, 4 ....3 5–9............4 10–14.........5 15–24.........6 25–29.........7 30–39.........8 40+...........9	a lot ....1 some ....2 not at all ....3 (uncertain) 4	3	4
than 2 wks......1 s < 1 mth ......2 h < 6 mths ......3 ns < 1 yr ....4 < 5 yrs............5 < 10 yrs ....6 s or more 7		3	4	1..............1 2..............2 3, 4 ....3 5–9............4 10–14.........5 15–24.........6 25–29.........7 30–39.........8 40+...........9	a lot ....1 some ....2 not at all ....3 (uncertain) 4	3	4
than 2 wks......1 s < 1 mth ......2 h < 6 mths ......3 ns < 1 yr ....4 < 5 yrs............5 < 10 yrs ....6 s or more 7		3	4	1..............1 2..............2 3, 4 ....3 5–9............4 10–14.........5 15–24.........6 25–29.........7 30–39.........8 40+...........9	a lot ....1 some ....2 not at all ....3 (uncertain) 4	3	4

RT ALL PRESCRIBED MEDICINES AT NEXT TABLE IF NO PRESCRIBED MEDICINES TAKEN GO TO Q.20

ASK ABOUT ALL PRESCRIBED MEDICINES

Now can we talk about _____
INSERT TYPE/NO AND
LETTER

	1	2	3	4	5	6
10. How long ago did you first get a prescription for _____ ?						
< 2 weeks	1	1	1	1	1	1
2 wks < 1 mth	2	2	2	2	2	2
1 mth < 6 mths	3	3	3	3	3	3
6mths < 1 yr	4	4	4	4	4	4
1 yr < 5 yrs	5	5	5	5	5	5
5 yrs < 10 yrs	6	6	6	6	6	6
10 yrs or more	7	7	7	7	7	7
11. How many prescriptions for _____ have you had altogether?						
1	1	1	1	1	1	1
2	2	2	2	2	2	2
3	3	3	3	3	3	3
4	4	4	4	4	4	4
5–9	5	5	5	5	5	5
10–19	6	6	6	6	6	6
20–39	7	7	7	7	7	7
40+	8	8	8	8	8	8
If one only skip to Q.14						
12. When was the last time you got a prescription for _____ ?						
< 2 wks	1	1	1	1	1	1
2 wks < 1 mth	2	2	2	2	2	2
1 mth < 6 mths	3	3	3	3	3	3
6 mths < 1 yr	4	4	4	4	4	4
1 yr < 5 yrs	5	5	5	5	5	5
5 yrs < 10 yrs	6	6	6	6	6	6
10 yrs or more	7	7	7	7	7	7
13. When you get a repeat prescription for _____ do you usually see the doctor or not?						
Always do	1	1	1	1	1	1
Usually do	2	2	2	2	2	2
Half and half	3	3	3	3	3	3
Usually do not	4	4	4	4	4	4

If (2, 3 or 4)
Can you tell me about the arrangements
for getting a repeat prescription without
seeing the doctor.

	I	2	3	4	5	6
INSERT TYPE/NO AND LETTER						

14. Would you say you take this medicine:

	I	2	3	4	5	6
Rather more than advised	I	I	I	I	I	I
Rather less than advised	2	2	2	2	2	2
Exactly as advised	3	3	3	3	3	3
or Have you not been advised how often and how much to take	4	4	4	4	4	4

If (*1 or 2*)
Why is that?

15. Is there anything about the medicine that makes it unpleasant or difficult to take/use?

	I	2	3	4	5	6
Yes	I	I	I	I	I	I
No	2	2	2	2	2	2

If YES (*1*) Can you tell me why?

16. Has anyone told you whether _____ has any side effects or whether after taking it you shouldn't drink alcohol, drive a car, eat certain things or take other drugs, or anything like that?

	I	2	3	4	5	6
Yes	I	I	I	I	I	I
No	2	2	2	2	2	2

If YES (*1*) Who told you?
What did they say?

17. Are any instructions about how often and how much to use, written on the medicine?

	I	2	3	4	5	6
Yes	I	I	I	I	I	I
No	2	2	2	2	2	2

18. Is the name of the drug written on it?

	I	2	3	4	5	6
Yes	3	3	3	3	3	3
No	4	4	4	4	4	4

If YES (*3*) *check*

19. Have any of your friends or relatives taken any of it?

	I	2	3	4	5	6
Yes	I	I	I	I	I	I
No	2	2	2	2	2	2

If YES (*1*) *Probe for details*

RETURN TO Q.10 FOR EACH PRESCRIBED MEDICINE

20. I'd now like to ask you about things you might have had wrong with you in the last two weeks.

Now can we talk about each one

What about:	Yes	No	Insert Symptom and Number indicate if arose at 32 or 33	Is _____ connected with any of your other symptoms? *List Numbers*	What do you think is the cause? *If injury* How did it happen?
1. Sore throat	1	o			
2. Breathlessness	2	o			
3. Coughs, catarrh or phlegm	3	o			
4. Cold, 'flu or running nose	4	o			
5. Constipation	5	o			
6. Diarrhoea	6	o			
7. Vomiting	7	o			
8. Indigestion	8	o			
9. Eye strain or other eye trouble	9	o			
10. Ear trouble	1	o			
11. Faintness or dizziness	2	o			
12. Headaches	3	o			
13. Pain or trouble passing water	4	o			
14. Loss of appetite	5	o			
15. Any problem being under- or over-weight	6	o			
16. Nerves, depression or irritability	7	o			
17. Pains in the chest	8	o			
18. Backache or pains in the back	9	o			
19. Aches or pains in the joints, muscles, legs or arms	1	o			
20. Palpitations or thumping heart	2	o			
21. Piles	3	o			
22. Sores or ulcers	4	o			
23. Rashes, itches or other skin troubles	5	o			
24. Sleeplessness	6	o			
25. Swollen ankles	7	o			
26. Burns, bruises, cuts or other accidents	8	o			
27. Trouble with teeth or gums	9	o			
28. Undue tiredness	1	o			
29. Corns, bunions or any trouble with your feet	2	o			
30. (Women's complaints like period pain)	3	o			
31. A temperature	4	o			
32. Any other symptoms that I haven't already mentioned? What?	5	o			
33. Can I check whether you've had any other symptoms related to bronchitis, hay fever, asthma, any other allergy, varicose veins, heart trouble, infectious diseases, rheumatism, arthritis or anything else? What?	6	o			

LIST ALL SYMPTOMS AT TABLE

Appendix VIII

ow long have you d _____? RTICULAR SYMPTOM <6mths <1yr $1-5$yr $5-10$yr 10yr+	Check. Now I think you said you had/had not taken something for _____ in the last two weeks. If taken nothing (2)		
	Yes	No	Can you tell me why not?
1 2 3 4 5 6	1	2	
1 2 3 4 5 6	1	2	
1 2 3 4 5 6	1	2	
1 2 3 4 5 6	1	2	
1 2 3 4 5 6	1	2	
1 2 3 4 5 6	1	2	
1 2 3 4 5 6	1	2	
1 2 3 4 5 6	1	2	
1 2 3 4 5 6	1	2	
1 2 3 4 5 6	1	2	
1 2 3 4 5 6	1	2	
1 2 3 4 5 6	1	2	
1 2 3 4 5 6	1	2	
1 2 3 4 5 6	1	2	
1 2 3 4 5 6	1	2	

ANY ADDITIONAL MEDICINES TAKEN CROP UP GO BACK TO Q.9 AND OBTAIN DETAILS

155

21. In the last two weeks have you consulted, either by telephoning or seeing, your general practitioner, his partners or locum, another general practitioner, a doctor at a hospital or any other doctor at all?
Yes 1   No 2
If YES (1) How many times? _____ *Go to Table*
If NO (2) Skip to Q.31
If More than Once

22. Can we talk about the first time in the last two weeks first.
Ask for Each Consultation

	1	2	3
23. Was it in the last seven days or the week before that? Last week	1	1	1
Week before	2	2	2
24. What illness or condition was it for? Anything else?			
25. Was that the first time you had seen Yes	3	3	3
a doctor for that (those conditions)? No	4	4	4
If No (4) How many times had you seen a doctor before about that 1	1	1	1
(those)? 2	2	2	2
3, 4	3	3	3
5–9	4	4	4
10+	5	5	5
If First Time Did you try anything yourself before going to the doctor? Yes	1	1	1
No	2	2	2
If Yes (1) What was that?			
26. Where did you see the doctor? Home	1	1	1
Surgery	2	2	2
Hospital OP	3	3	3
Telephone	4	4	4
Other (specify)	5	5	5
27. Whom did you see? Own G.P.	1	1	1
Partner	2	2	2
Locum	3	3	3
Other G.P.	4	4	4
Hospital Dr	5	5	5
Other (specify)	6	6	6
28. Was there anything else you would have liked to talk to the doctor about Yes	1	1	1
if he'd had plenty of time? No	2	2	2
If YES (1) What was that?			
29. Did the doctor do any of these things: Give you an examination or check-up	1	1	1
Refer you to a hospital or anywhere else	2	2	2
Give you any treatment himself	3	3	3
Give you any other advice or reassurance	4	4	4
Give you a medical certificate	5	5	5
None of these	6	6	6
30. Did the doctor give you a prescription or medicine? Yes	3	3	3
No	4	4	4
If YES (3) For how many things?			

Return to Q.23 for Each Consultation

Appendix VIII

31. *To All.* In the last two weeks have you got a prescription either by phoning up, writing for it, getting a repeat from the doctor's receptionist or in any other way that did not involve seeing the doctor, or any prescriptions from the dentist? Yes......1 No 2
    If YES (1)
    (a) How many? ——————

    If YES (1) Can you tell me how you got it (them)?

Ask	Got
Post	Post 1
Post	Call 2
Call	Call 3
Call	Post......4
Phone	Post......5
Phone	Call 6
	Dentist 7
	Other (specify)......8

32. Were there any other prescriptions you were given that you did not necessarily get made up or take? Yes......1   No 2
    If YES (1) Check that they are recorded above

33. Now can I check. In the last two weeks you have been given _____ prescriptions. *Check that those mentioned at Qs 10, 12, 30 are included.*

If no prescriptions at Qs 30, 31, 32 skip to Q.39

Ask for Each Prescription Can we talk about the one you got when (DESCRIPTIONS OF CIRCUMSTANCES)	1	2	3
34. What was the medicine?			
35. Did you get the prescription made up or not? Yes	1	1	1
If NO (2) Can you tell me why? No	2	2	2
Skip to Q.39			
36. Did you pay the 2/6 prescription 2/6	3	3	3
charge or not or did you pay nothing	4	4	4
for the medicine itself? medicine	5	5	5
If (5) How much was that?			
37. When you got the prescription made up did you try it? Yes	1	1	1
If NO (2) Why not? No	2	2	2
38. Have you still got some of it? Yes	3	3	3
No	4	4	4
If YES (3) Are you still taking it? Yes	5	5	5
No	6	6	6
Probe about where left overs are thrown away *If YES (5) What will you do with any that is left?*			
If NO (6) What have you done with what is left?			
If NO (4) Have you used it all up or thrown it away or what?			

Return to Q.34 for Each Prescription

157

39. Do you go out to work?
    Yes.................................... 1
    No 2
    If YES (1)
    Have you had any time off work
    because of illness in the last
    two weeks?
    Yes.................................... 3
    No 4
    If YES (3)
    How many days?

	Off work	In bed
$\frac{1}{2}$ or 1 day	1	1
2–4 days	2	2
5–7 days	3	3
8 < whole time	4	4
All time	5	5

40. Have you had any days in bed
    because of illness in the last
    two weeks?
    Code Above

41. Can you give me some
    estimate of how many times in
    the last year you have consulted
    a general practitioner?
    Not at all 0
    Once 1
    2–4 2
    5–9 3
    10+ 4

42. When was the last most recent
    time you consulted a general
    practitioner?
    < 2 weeks 1
    2 wks < 1 month 2
    1 mth < 6 mths 3
    6 mths < 1 year 4
    1 year < 5 years 5
    5 years < 10 years 6
    10 years or more 7

43. Which is the quickest and
    easiest to get to: your doctor's
    surgery or a chemist shop?
    Surgery 1
    Chemist............................ 2
    Same 3

44. How long does it generally take
    you to get to your doctor's
    surgery?
    Less than 15 mins 1
    15 mins < 30 mins 2
    30 mins < 45 mins............. 3
    45 mins < 1 hour 4
    1 hour or more 5

45. How long do you generally
    have to wait at the surgery?
    Less than 15 mins 1
    15 mins < 30 mins............. 2
    30 mins < 45 mins............. 3
    45 mins < 1 hour 4
    1 hour < 1$\frac{1}{2}$ hours 5
    1$\frac{1}{2}$ hours < 2 hours 6
    2 hours or more 7

46. Do you think the time it takes
    you to get to the doctor or the
    time you have to wait sometimes
    discourages you from going to
    the doctor?
    Yes.................................... 1
    No 2
    If YES (1) Does this mean you
    don't consult at all or that you
    ask him to visit or what?
    Don't go 3
    Ask him to visit 4
    Other (specify) 5
    If DON'T GO (3) What was
    the matter with you the last
    time this happened?

47. When you go to your doctor do
    you feel he has enough time to
    listen to you and do all that is
    necessary or not?
    Yes.................................... 1
    No 2
    If NO (2) In what way?

48. If you could have ten minutes
    uninterrupted discussion either
    with your doctor or with
    another doctor you found
    sympathetic is there anything
    particular you would like to ask
    them about?
    Yes.................................... 1
    No 2
    If YES (1) What is it?

49. If you were worried about a personal problem that wasn't strictly a medical one, do you think you might discuss it with your doctor?

Yes............................... 1
No 2
Uncertain 3
Why is that?

50. Here are some statements about doctors, could you tell me whether you agree, disagree or feel neutral about them?

	Ag.	N.	Dis.
(a) The less you see of doctors, the better for your health.	1	2	3
(b) A person understands his own health better than most doctors do.	4	5	6

51. Do you agree, disagree or feel neutral about the following statements?

	Ag.	N.	Dis.
(a) Making sure your bowels open every day is important for keeping healthy.	1	2	3
(b) It is only sensible to take aspirins or something like that whenever you get a headache.	4	5	6

52. I am going to read a short list of people and things which may influence peoples' knowledge about treatment of illness. Will you tell me whether you think you have learnt anything about treatment of illness from:

	Yes	No	Most
Television	1	o	1
Your parents	2	o	2
Other relatives	3	o	3
Your general practitioner	4	o	4
Other doctors	5	o	5
Radio	6	o	6
Friends or neighbours	7	o	7
Newspapers, magazines, books	8	o	8
Health visitors or other nurses	9	o	9
Anywhere or anyone else (specify)	y	o	y

If Other Relatives—Who?
(a) Which of those do you think has been most helpful?
    Code Above
(b) Can you give me some idea of the sort of things you have learnt from them?

53. Here is a series of twelve questions. Would you please answer, yes or no, and try not to think too long about the exact meaning of them.

	Yes	No	D.K.
(a) Do you like plenty of excitement and bustle around you?	1	2	3
(b) Does your mood often go up and down?	1	2	3
(c) Are you rather lively?	1	2	3

Continued overleaf

Appendix VIII

	Yes	No	D.K.
(d) Do you ever feel 'just miserable' for no good reason?	1	2	3
(e) Do you like mixing with people?	1	2	3
(f) When you get annoyed do you need someone friendly to talk to about it?	1	2	3
(g) Would you call yourself happy-go-lucky?	1	2	3
(h) Are you often troubled about feelings of guilt?	1	2	3

	Yes	No	D.K.
(i) Can you usually let yourself go and enjoy yourself a lot at a gay party?	1	2	3
(j) Would you call yourself tense or 'highly strung'?	1	2	3
(k) Do you like practical jokes?	1	2	3
(l) Do you suffer from sleeplessness?	1	2	3

Explain: Those are the only questions like that. Please think carefully about the rest of the questions I'd like to ask you.

54. I have a list of conditions or symptoms which I will read to you. I would like you to try and imagine what you would do for each. Would you consult the doctor, do something yourself or what would you do—or wouldn't you do anything?

	Consult doctor	Treat yourself	Other (specify)	Nothing
A constant feeling of depression for about three weeks	1 *Comments*	2	3	0
Difficulty in sleeping for about a week	1 *Comments*	2	3	0
A heavy cold with a temperature and running nose	1 *Comments*	2	3	0
A headache more than once a week for a month	1 *Comments*	2	3	0
A very sore throat for three days and no other symptoms	1 *Comments*	2	3	0
A boil that doesn't clear up in a week	1 *Comments*	2	3	0

160

55. There are some things that doctors can cure completely, others that they can make feel better and some that they can do very little about. Do you think they can generally cure, help, or not help:

	Cure	Help	Not help	DK	Comments
Rheumatism	1	2	3	4	
A bad cold	1	2	3	4	
Corns	1	2	3	4	
Skin cancer	1	2	3	4	
Arthritis	1	2	3	4	
Depression	1	2	3	4	
Sleeplessness	1	2	3	4	
Frequent headaches	1	2	3	4	
Bronchitis	1	2	3	4	

56. Which of these illnesses do you think it is possible to catch from someone else?

Diabetes	Yes	1
	No	2
	(D.K.)..............	3
Polio	Yes	4
	No..................	5
	(D.K.)..............	6
Bronchitis	Yes	7
	No..................	8
	(D.K.)..............	9
T.B.	Yes	1
	No..................	2
	(D.K.)..............	3
Anaemia	Yes	4
	No..................	5
	(D.K.)..............	6

57. In general do you think a chemist is a good person to ask for advice when you are not feeling well?

Yes 1
No.................. 2

Can you tell me why?

58. Do you smoke cigarettes?

Yes 1
No.................. 2

If YES (1)

I. How many manufactured cigarettes do you usually smoke?
(a) per working day _____
(b) at weekends _____

II. How much tobacco (oz) do you normally smoke per week in hand-rolled cigarettes? _____

CLASSIFICATION
As I explained before we don't use any names in our study but we do like to know one or two things about the people we interview.

59. How old are you?

21–24 1
25–34.............................. 2
35–44.............................. 3
45–54.............................. 4
55–64.............................. 5
65–74.............................. 6
75+ 7

60. Are you:

    Single............................ 1
    Married 2
    Widowed.......................... 3
    Divorced.......................... 4
    Separated......................... 5

61. Sex:

    Male 1
    Female............................ 2

62. *If Man or Single Woman Under 65*
Could you tell me your occupation?

    If Man or Single Woman Over 65
    What was your main occupation?

    If Married Women or Widow
    What is (was) your husband's
    (main) occupation?

    Self-employed with employees 1
    Self-employed without
       employees 2
    Manager 3
    Foreman 4
    Other employee 5

63. How old were you when you left
school?

    14 or less 1
    15................................... 2
    16................................... 3
    17 or more 4

64. Have you had any further education
or training?

    Yes 8
    No 9
    If YES (8) What/Where?
    University......................... 1
    Training College 2
    Technical College 3
    Secretarial........................ 4
    Apprenticeship................... 5
    Other (specify).................. 6

65. Can you tell me about all the
people in this household?

Relationship to subject	Sex		Age group			
	M	F	under 15	15–44	45–65	65+
1 SUBJECT	1	2	3	4	5	6
2		1	2	3	4	5	6
3	1	2	3	4	5	6
4	1	2	3	4	5	6
5	1	2	3	4	5	6
6	1	2	3	4	5	6
7	1	2	3	4	5	6
8	1	2	3	4	5	6
9	1	2	3	4	5	6
10	1	2	3	4	5	6
11	1	2	3	4	5	6

Check So there are _____ of you
altogether.

66. Are you on the telephone?

    Yes.................................. 1
    No 2

67. Have you (has someone in this
household) got a car?

    Yes.................................. 3
    No 4

*If respondent had a prescription in
the two weeks before interview,
(Check with Page 7)*

68. Would you be willing to keep a
diary about all the medicines you
take during the next two weeks?
We will give you ten shillings for
doing it.

    Yes.................................. 1
    No 2

*Leave a stamped addressed envelope
and give instructions to post diary
after fourteen days.*

Appendix VIII

69. *Check* I think you said you:

remembered getting a letter
from us 1
did not get a letter from us.... 2
If (1)
Do you think the letter was
helpful or would you have
preferred me just to call without
sending a letter first, or don't
you mind?
Prefer letter......................... 1
Prefer just to call.................. 2
Don't mind 3

*If marked X on sample list and there
are children in the household under fifteen
ask the mother of the children the questions
on the other two questionnaires (2 and 3).*

*If marked X on sample list and there are
no children in the household under fifteen ask
the informant, or if he is a married man,
his wife the questions on questionnaire 3.*

*If not marked X on sample list or if
informant is not answering questions on
questionnaires 2 and 3 thank them and
leave the survey leaflet. Check whether they
want to ask you any questions about the
Survey or the Institute.*

Length of interview
Less than 30 mins 1
30 < 45................................. 2
45 < 60................................. 3
60 < 75................................. 4
75 < 90................................. 5
90 < 120............................... 6
120+ 7

Date of interview

Interviewer

Respondent on questionnaire 2
Insert number from household table

Respondent on Questionnaire 3

Postal questionnaire to general practitioners

MEDICINES SURVEY

Please tick your answers where appropriate

1. Are there any kinds of drugs
that are only obtainable on
prescription at the moment that
you would like to see made freely
available to the public?
Yes.........
No.........
If YES—What kinds? Why?

2. Are there any kinds of drugs freely
obtainable that you would like to
see made available on prescription
only?
Yes.........
No.........
If YES What kinds? Why?

3. What proportion, if any, of your
consultations would you estimate
are for ailments that people could
treat or cope with themselves
without seeing the doctor?

90% or more   ....
75% but less than 90%.........
50% but less than 75%.........
25% but less than 50%.........
10% but less than 25%.........
5% but less than 10% ....
Less than 5%   ....
None   ....

4. Which of the following ailments do you think are generally suitable for most adults to treat themselves without consulting a doctor?
   (*a*) A constant feeling of depression for about three weeks.........
   (*b*) Difficulty in sleeping for about a week.........
   (*c*) A heavy cold with a temperature and running nose.........
   (*d*) A headache more than once a week for a month.........
   (*e*) A very sore throat for three days and no other symptoms.........
   (*f*) A boil that does not clear up in a week.........

5. At two-thirds of the consultations reported on our study patients said they had been given a prescription. Do you think you give prescriptions:
   At more consultations than this.........
   At fewer consultations than this.........
   or At about the same proportion.........

6. Do you do anything to encourage appropriate self-treatment among your patients?
   Yes.........
   No.........
   If YES What?

7. Do you do anything to discourage inappropriate self treatment among your patients?
   Yes.........
   No.........
   If YES What?

8. One-fifth of the prescriptions the people on our study had had during a two-week period had been obtained without seeing the doctor. Do you think the proportion of prescriptions you sign without seeing the patients is more, less or about the same as this?
   More than this.........
   Less than this.........
   About the same.........

9. What arrangements, if any, are there for your patients who need repeat prescriptions?

10. Which drugs, if any, are most commonly obtained on repeat prescriptions by your patients without seeing you?

11. How often do you reckon to see patients for whom you have prescribed oral contraceptives?
    At least every 3 months.........
    every 6 months.........
    once a year.........
    Other, please say what.........

12. How often do you reckon to see patients for whom you prescribe sleeping tablets for insomnia?
    At least once a month.........
    every 3 months.........
    every 6 months.........
    once a year.........
    Other, please say what.........

13. How many times during the last two weeks have you suggested that a patient buys medicine, tablets or ointment from the chemist without a prescription? What sort of medicines?

14. If you had more time to spend with each patient do you think you would give:
    Fewer prescriptions.........
    More prescriptions.........
    The same number.........

15. If you had more time do you think your prescribing would change in other ways, for example, the types of drugs or the quantities you prescribe?

16. As you know the amount of prescribing varies from one part of the country to another. What do you think is the main reason for this?
    Different levels of sickness.........
    Different habits and attitudes of patients.........
    Different prescribing practices of general practitioners.........
    Something else? What?.........

17. Do you think the general public ought to be encouraged to ask the pharmacist questions about health and medicine or not?
    Yes.........
    No.........

18. Do you think the general public ought to be encouraged to ask health visitors and other nurses questions about health and medicines or not?
    Yes.........
    No.........

19. About how many drug firms' representatives have you seen in the last four weeks?
    None.........
    1–4.........
    5–9.........
    10 or more.........

20. Please tick in the first column *all* sources of information that you find useful for learning about new drugs put on the market, and in the second column the *single* source you find most useful.

	All helpful sources	One most helpful
Medical Journals		
Drug firm literature		
Drug firm representatives		
MIMS		
B.N.F.		
Prescribers' Journal		
Letters from hospital consultants		
Discussion with other doctors		
Local clinical meetings		
Local drug firm meetings		
Refresher courses		
Anything else (SPECIFY):		

21. Do you think anything should be done to try and reduce the number of consultations which patients make for minor ailments which are self-limiting and can be self treated?
    What?

Finally a few details about your practice:

22. Is your practice:
    Single handed.........
    Self and assistant.........
    Self and partner
    Self and two others.........
    Self and three or more others.........

23. Do you have an appointment system at:
    All surgeries.........
    Some surgeries.........
    Or none of them.........

24. What is the approximate number of your N.H.S. patients? If you are in partnership please estimate the number you yourself look after.
    Under 1,500.........
    1,500–1,999.........
    2,000–2,499.........
    2,500–2,999.........
    3,000–3,499.........
    3,500 or more.........

25. Do you hold any paid or honorary appointment on the staff of any N.H.S. hospital? (i.e. as a consultant, clinical assistant or other grade of medical officer)?
    Yes.........
    No.........

26. Do you do your own dispensing?
    Yes.........
    No.........

27. Have you any other comments or suggestions to make about medication in the National Health context?
    THANK YOU FOR YOUR HELP
    If you would like to discuss anything personally please put a tick here ☐ and we will make an appointment either to visit or telephone you.
    If you would like to be informed about the final results of the survey please put a tick here ☐

REFERENCES

Advertising Association, 1962, *Advertising of Vitamin Products.*

ALDERSON, M. R., 1970, 'Social class and the health service', *Medical Officer*, Vol. CXXIV, 50–2.

Association of the British Pharmaceutical Industry, 1970, *The Pharmaceutical Industry and the Nation's Health* (fifth ed.).

Automobile Association, 1969, 'The drugged driver', *Drive*, new year issue.

BALINT, M., HUNT, J., JOYCE, D., MARINKER, M. and WOODCOCK, J., 1970, *Treatment or Diagnosis*, London, Tavistock.

BEECHER, H. K., 1955, 'The powerful placebo', *Journal of the American Medical Association*, Vol. 159, 1,602–6.

BONNAR, J., GOLDBERG, A. and SMITH, J. A., 1969, 'Do pregnant women take their iron?', *Lancet*, i, 457–8.

BRADSHAW, S., 1966, *The Drugs You Take*, London, Hutchinson.

CARTWRIGHT, ANN, 1957, 'The effect of obtaining information from different informants on a family morbidity inquiry', *Applied Statistics*, Vol. 6, 18–25.

CARTWRIGHT, ANN, 1959, 'Some problems in the collection and analysis of morbidity data obtained from sample surveys', *Millbank Memorial Fund Quarterly*, Vol. 37, 343–8.

CARTWRIGHT, ANN, 1967, *Patients and their Doctors*, London, Routledge & Kegan Paul.

CARTWRIGHT, ANN, 1968, 'General practitioners and family planning', *Medical Officer*, Vol. CXX, 43–6.

CARTWRIGHT, ANN, 1970, *Parents and Family Planning Services*, London, Routledge & Kegan Paul.

CARTWRIGHT, ANN, HOCKEY, LISBETH and ANDERSON, J. L., *Life Before Death* (in press).

CLARKE, MAY, 1969, *Trouble with Feet*, Occasional Papers in Social Administration No. 29, London, G. Bell.

COCHRANE, A. L. and MOORE, F., 1971, 'Expected and observed values for the prescription of vitamin B_{12} in England and Wales', *British Journal of Preventive and Social Medicine*, Vol. 25, 147–51.

Code of Advertising Practice Committee, 1970, *The British Code of Advertising Practice* (fourth ed.).

CONNELL, A. M., HILTON, C., IRVINE, G., LENNARD JONES, J. E. and MISIEWICZ, J. J., 1965, 'Variation of bowel habit in two population samples', *British Medical Journal*, ii, 1095–9.

Department of Health and Social Security, 1969, *Annual Report for 1968* HMSO.

DOUGLAS, J. W. B. and BLOMFIELD, J. M., 1958, *Children under Five*, London, Allen & Unwin.

EASTWOOD, M. R. and TREVELYAN, M. H., 1971, 'Smoking and neurotic illness', *Lancet*, i, 107–8.

References

ELDER, RUTH, and ACHESON, ROY M., 1970, New Haven Survey of Joint Diseases, XIV, 'Social class and behaviour in response to symptoms of osteoarthrosis', *Millbank Memorial Fund Quarterly*, Vol. XLVIII, No. 4, Pt. 1, 449–502.

EYSENCK, H. J., *Smoking, Health and Personality*, London, Weidenfeld & Nicolson.

EYSENCK, S. B. G. and EYSENCK, H. J., 1964, 'An improved short questionnaire for the measurement of extraversion and neuroticism', *Life Sciences*, Vol. 3, 1103–9.

General Register Office, 1960 and 1967, *The Registrar-General's statistical review of England and Wales*, Part 1, Tables, Medical, HMSO.

General Register Office, 1966, *Classification of Occupations*, HMSO.

General Register Office, 1967, *Sample Census 1966*, HMSO.

GLASSER, M. A., 1958, 'A study of the public's acceptance of the Salk vaccine program', *American Journal of Public Health*, 48, 141–6.

GRAY, P. G. and CARTWRIGHT, ANN, 1954, 'Who gets the medicine?', *Applied Statistics*, Vol. III, 19–28.

GRAY, P. G. and CORLETT, T., 1951, 'Sampling for the Social Survey', *Journal of the Royal Statistical Society*, Series A. CXIII, Part II, 150–99.

HORDER, J. and HORDER, E., 1954, 'Illness in general practice', *Practitioner*, 173, 177–87.

JEFFERYS, MARGOT, BROTHERSTON, J. H. F. and CARTWRIGHT, ANN, 1960, 'Consumption of medicines on a working-class housing estate', *British Journal of Preventive and Social Medicine*, Vol. 14, 64–76.

JOYCE, C. R. B., 'Quantitative estimates of dependence on the symbolic function of drugs' in Steinberg, H. (ed.), 1969, *Scientific Basis of Drug Dependence*, London, Churchill.

JOYCE, C. R. B., LAST, J. M. and WEATHERALL, M., 1968, 'Personal factors as a cause of differences in prescribing by general practitioners', *British Journal of Preventive and Social Medicine*, Vol. 22, 170–7.

KALIMO, E., 1969, *Determinants of Medical Care Utilisation*, National Pensions Institute, Finland.

KESSEL, N. and SHEPHERD, M., 1965, 'The health and attitudes of people who seldom consult a doctor', *Medical Care*, Vol. 3, 6–10.

KOSA, J., ALPERT, J. J. and HAGGERTY, R. J., 1967, 'On the reliability of family health information. A comparative study of mothers' reports on illness and related behaviour', *Social Science and Medicine*, Vol. 1, 165–81.

LANCE, HILARY, 1971, 'Transport services in general practice', Supplement of the *Journal of the Royal College of General Practitioners*, Vol. 21, No. 3.

Lancet editorial, 1970, 'Control of drugs', *Lancet*, 21 March.

LINNETT, M., 1968, 'Prescribing habits in general practice', *Proceedings of the Royal Society of Medicine*, Vol. 61, 613–15.

LOGAN, W. P. D. and BROOKE, E. M., 1957, *The Survey of Sickness, 1943 to 1952*, General Register Office Studies on Medical and Population Subjects, No. 12, HMSO.

MADDOCK, D. H., 1971, Master's thesis for Welsh School of Pharmacy reported in *Guardian*, 19 April.

MARTIN, J. P., 1957, *Social Aspects of Prescribing*, London, Heinemann.

167

References

MECHANIC, D., 1970, 'Correlates of frustration among British general practitioners', *Journal of Health and Social Behaviour*, Vol. II, 87–104.

Ministry of Health, 1962–1967, *Annual Reports*, HMSO.

National Opinion Polls Ltd, 1965, *Home medication survey*, NOP 1470.

NICHOLSON, W. A., 1967, 'Collection of unwanted drugs from private homes', *British Medical Journal*, iii, 730–1.

Office of Health Economics, 1968, *Without Prescription*.

Office of Health Economics, 1971, *Off Sick*.

PARISH, PETER A., 1971, 'The prescribing of psychotropic drugs in general practice', Supplement of the *Journal of the Royal College of General Practitioners*, Vol. 21, No. 4.

Registrar-General, 1968, *Statistical Review of England and Wales for the Year 1967*, Part 1, *Tables, Medical*, HMSO.

REID, J. J. A., 1956, 'Regular use of laxatives by school children', *British Medical Journal*, ii, 25–7.

REIN, MARTIN, 1969, 'Social class and the health service', *New Society*, Vol. 14, 807–10.

ROBINSON, DAVID, 1971, *The Process of Becoming Ill*, London, Routledge & Kegan Paul.

Royal College of General Practitioners, 1970, *Present State and Future Needs of General Practice* (second ed.), Council of the Royal College of General Practitioners.

SAMORA, J., SAUNDERS, L. and LARSON, R. F., 1961, 'Medical vocabulary knowledge among hospital patients', *Journal of Health and Human Behaviour*, Vol. 2, 83–92.

SAMORA, J., SAUNDERS, L. and LARSON, R. F., 1962, 'Knowledge about specific diseases in four selected samples', *Journal of Health and Human Behaviour*, Vol. 3, 176–85.

Scottish Home and Health Department, 1969, *Health and Welfare Services in Scotland, Report for 1968*, Edinburgh, HMSO.

SILVERMAN, C., 1968, *The Epidemiology of Depression*, Baltimore, Johns Hopkins Press.

STOCKS, P., 1949, *Sickness in the Population of England and Wales in 1944–47*, General Register Office Studies on Medical and Population Subjects, No. 2, HMSO.

TITMUSS, R. M., 1968, *Commitment to Welfare*, London, Allen & Unwin.

TODD, R. G. (ed.), 1967, *Extra Pharmacopoeia Martindale* (twenty-fifth ed.), London, Pharmaceutical Press.

TOWNSEND, PETER and WEDDERBURN, DOROTHY, 1965, *The Aged in the Welfare State*, Occasional Papers on Social Administration, No. 14, London, G. Bell.

WADSWORTH, M. E. J., BUTTERFIELD, W. J. H. and BLANEY, R., 1971, *Health and Sickness: the Choice of Treatment*, London, Tavistock.

WALLER, JANE, 1971, 'Some factors associated with use of medical services for a trivial condition', Paper presented at the Sixth Meeting of the International Epidemiological Association.

WATERS, W. E., 1971, 'Smoking and neuroticism', *British Journal of Preventive and Social Medicine*, Vol. 25, 162–4.

References

WHITFIELD, M., 1968, 'The pharmacists' contribution to medical care', *Practitioner*, Vol. 200, 434–8.

WILSON, J. D. and ENOCH, M. D., 1967, 'Estimation of drug rejection by schizophrenic in-patients with analysis of clinical factors', *British Journal of Psychiatry*, Vol. 113, 209–11.

WILLIAMSON, J., 1967, 'Detecting disease in clinical geriatrics' *Gerontologia Clinica*, Vol. 9, 236–42.

WOOLF, MYRA, 1971, *Family Intentions*, HMSO.

INDEX

Index

Index

Liverpool–Walton, study area, 3, 124–5, 128, 140
Living room, medicines kept in, 86–8
Local authorities
collection of unused medicines, 81
health education by, 67
Logan, W. P. D., 6n
Lower respiratory preparations, 23–9
and frequency, 40
hoarding, 91
in the home, 84–5
and repeat prescriptions, 44
waste of, 93

Maddock, D. H., 96n
Marinker, Marshall, 42n, 43n, 49n, 73n, 121n
Martin, J. P., 7n
Mechanic, David, 76n
Medicinal food and drink, 23–9, 138
and frequency, 40
in the home, 85
patterns in the use of, 109–11
Medicines, classifications of, 25–7, 83, 100, 105, 138–9
Medicines, number of (prescribed and non-prescribed), 13, 14
and age, 17, 18
in the home, 82–3
kept by different social classes, 86–7
kept in different areas, 88–9
kept in households of differing size and composition, 89–90
and neuroticism, 60
and number of symptoms, 14
and self-reliance, 58
and sex, 20–1
and social class, 52
and time of year, 140
Medicine taking in general, 1, 5, 6, 13–22, 117–19, 122
and doctors' response, 133–4
and faith in doctors, 59–60
and reliance on the doctor, 57
and self-reliance, 58
and symptom reporting, 101
see also Prescribed medication; Self-medication

Mental illness, 111
see also Depression; Nerves, depression or irritability
Merton and Morden, study area, 3, 124–5, 128
Middle class, see Social class
Migraine and analgesic use, 100
Ministry of Health, 1n
Misiewicz, J. J., 53n
Misuse of medicines, 46–7, 80–1, 120
Monthly Index of Medical Specialities, 25
source of information about drugs, 72
Moore, F., 110n
Mouth and throat preparations, 30, 138
see also Ear, nose and throat preparations
Musculo-skeletal symptoms, see Aches or pains in joints, muscles, legs, arms

Nappy rash, see Skin trouble
National Health Service, 1, 36, 94
National Opinion Polls Ltd, 7n
Nerves, depression or irritability, 11, 12, 122
and age, 16, 112–13
and medication, 33
and oral contraceptive use, 115
and sedative use, 111–13
and sex, 19, 20, 112
and social class, 113
Neuroticism, see Personality differences
New Forest, study area, 3, 124–5, 128, 140
Nicholson, W. A., 7n, 81n
Nurses, 68
advice to patients, 69–70, 97, 115
Nutritional, blood and metabolic preparations, 23–9
and frequency, 40
and repeat prescriptions, 43–4, 73
hoarding of, 91
in the home, 85
waste of, 93

and size of list, 75–6
and size of practice, 76–7
see also Repeat prescribing
Prescription charges, 34
Psychotropic drugs, 7, 121
see also Central nervous system
preparations; Sedatives; Anti-
depressants

Rashes, *see* Skin trouble
Receptionists, 118
Refresher courses, source of information about drugs, 72
Regions, stratification of sample by,
124–5
Register of Electors, 124
Registrar-General, 80n
Reid, J. J. A., 106n
Rein, Martin, 50n
Relatives, advice about self-medica-
tions, 13, 97–8, 105
Reliance on the doctor, 54–6
and doctors' response, 134
Repeat prescribing, 2, 41–5, 48, 121,
123
and social class, 52
without seeing the doctor, 72–3
Respiratory system remedies
doctors' views on, 73
in the home, 84–7
patterns in the use of, 107–9
recommended by doctors, 69
and repeat prescribing, 73
see also Ear, nose and throat preparations; Lower respiratory
preparations
Respiratory symptoms and diseases,
116
see also, Cold, 'flu or running nose;
Coughs, catarrh or phlegm
Response rate
of adults, 3–5, 124, 126
of doctors, 132–4
Restricted areas, 131
and doctors' response, 132–3
Rheumatic disease preparations,
23–9, 138
and frequency, 40

hoarding of, 91–2
in the home, 84–5
and repeat prescriptions, 44
waste of, 93
Rheumatism, 30
and analgesic use, 100–2
and health-salt use, 105
patients' views on doctors' ability
to cure, 59, 141
Robinson, David, 13n
Role perception, 121–2
Royal College of General Practitioners, 2n
Rural population in study areas, 125
see also Area differences
Rural practice payments
doctors in the sample, 131
response, 33

Samora, J., 53n
Sample
of adults, 3–4, 124–6, 146
of children, 4, 127–9
of general practitioners, 4, 130–7
of households, 4, 81, 126–8
Sampling errors, 144–5
Saunders, L., 53n
Scottish Home and Health Department, 5, 95n
Screening, 68
Season, *see* Time of year
Secretaries, *see* Receptionists
Sedatives, sleeping tablets and tranquillisers, 24, 139
in the home, 84
patterns in the use of, 111–14
and repeat prescriptions, 72
and reweighting for bias, 147
and sleeplessness, 115–16
and social class, 52
see also Central nervous system
preparations
Self-medication, 2, 30, 120
and age, 17, 18
and bias in the sample, 126
doctors encourage and discourage,
68
and doctors' response, 133–4

Index

patients' views on doctors' ability
to cure, 59, 141
predicted action for, 55, 65–6, 118
and sedative use, 111–13, 115–16
and sex, 20, 112
and social class, 113
Slimming preparations, 24
and frequency, 40
and repeat prescriptions, 44
see also Nutritional, blood and
metabolic preparations
Smith, J. A., 46n
Smoking
giving up, 68, 116
and personality, 143
and sex differences, 107
and symptom reporting, 107–8,
116
Social class, 50–3
classification of, 146–7
and consumption of medicines, 31
and discussion of personal problems with doctor, 56
and knowledge, 53–4
and laxative use, 106
and medicines in the home, 86–9
and reliance on the doctor, 55–6
sampling error, 144–5
and sedative use, 113
and study areas, 125
and symptom reporting, 113
and time of year interviewed, 140
Sore throat, 11, 15, 30
and age, 16, 101
and analgesic use, 100–1
doctors' views on self-treatment
for, 65–6
and medication, 33
predicted action for, 55, 65–6
and season, 107
Sores, ulcers, 11
and age, 16
and sex, 20
and sum preparation use, 103
Southampton–Itchen, study area, 3,
124–5, 128, 140
Spouse, advice on self-medication,
98

Stability, *see* Personality differences
Statistical significance, 144–5
Stimulants, *see* Anti-depressants;
Central nervous system preparations
Stocks, P., 13n
Stroke, 111
Study areas
selection of, 124
social class and sampling error, 143
Suicide, 80
Sulphonamides, *see* Antibiotics, anti-
infective agents etc.
Suppositories, rectal preparations,
24
and frequency, 40
and repeat prescriptions, 44
see also Digestive system preparations
Surgery, general practitioner's
accessibility of, 96–7
Surgical clothing etc., 23–9
and frequency, 40
in the home, 85
and repeat prescriptions, 44–5
Survey of Sickness, 13
Symptoms, 10–12
and age, 15, 17, 18, 19
and medication, 30–6
and neuroticism, 60
number of, 8–9, 11, 13, 118
and position in the family, 61
and reliance on the doctor, 56
and reweighting for bias, 147
and sex, 19, 21
and social class, 50–2
and use of oral contraceptives, 115
Swansea–West, study area, 3, 124–5,
128, 140

Teeth, trouble with, 11, 12
and age, 16
and health rating, 10, 118
and sex, 20
Temperature, 11, 15
and age, 16
and health rating, 10
and sex, 20